PILLARS OF ASCENSION

TOOLS TO ACHIEVE YOUR BEST SELF,
EMOTIONALLY, SPIRITUALLY, AND PHYSICALLY

CANDY HOLMES-FOSTER

BALBOA.PRESS
A DIVISION OF HAY HOUSE

Copyright © 2024 Candy Holmes-Foster.

All rights reserved. No part of this book may be used or reproduced by any means, graphic, electronic, or mechanical, including photocopying, recording, taping or by any information storage retrieval system without the written permission of the author except in the case of brief quotations embodied in critical articles and reviews.

Balboa Press books may be ordered through booksellers or by contacting:

Balboa Press
A Division of Hay House
1663 Liberty Drive
Bloomington, IN 47403
www.balboapress.com
844-682-1282

Because of the dynamic nature of the Internet, any web addresses or links contained in this book may have changed since publication and may no longer be valid. The views expressed in this work are solely those of the author and do not necessarily reflect the views of the publisher, and the publisher hereby disclaims any responsibility for them.

The author of this book does not dispense medical advice or prescribe the use of any technique as a form of treatment for physical, emotional, or medical problems without the advice of a physician, either directly or indirectly. The intent of the author is only to offer information of a general nature to help you in your quest for emotional and spiritual well-being. In the event you use any of the information in this book for yourself, which is your constitutional right, the author and the publisher assume no responsibility for your actions.

Any people depicted in stock imagery provided by Getty Images are models, and such images are being used for illustrative purposes only.
Certain stock imagery © Getty Images.

Print information available on the last page.

ISBN: 979-8-7652-4761-7 (sc)
ISBN: 979-8-7652-4762-4 (hc)
ISBN: 979-8-7652-4760-0 (e)

Library of Congress Control Number: 2024901873

Balboa Press rev. date: 05/06/2024

For my husband, John
Thank you for believing unconditionally in me. I love you.

INTRODUCTION

My original vision for this book had three parts that converged. These three parts laid out the three pillars of holistic wellness—emotional, spiritual, and physical. I soon found that wasn't possible because these three pillars are so intertwined and connected. As I thought I was working on a physical aspect, it would naturally take on an emotional and spiritual tone. This totally makes sense if we are living with any kind of balance in these areas at all.

There is no perfect place to start this journey. It will look different for each and every one of us. No matter who you are or where you are starting from, I believe there is help among these pages. Some of you will come here physically strong. That will be the perfect starting point for you. From there, you can build on your emotional and spiritual strength and balance.

If you come here in a good emotional space, then that will help you build from there. If the spiritual space is where you are beginning, then that is your path. As you progress, each pillar will strengthen the others. So as you progress, notice that even though I've somewhat created three sections for these three pillars, the lines will blur and emerge with each other throughout, much like the journey itself.

Today I am thrilled to present the pages of this book to you. This is a project that I have contemplated for years and started repeatedly. This is the last time I will begin and the first time I will finish this dream of sharing my experiences and knowledge with the world.

Whether you are searching for a solution to any emotional, spiritual, or physical ailment, pain, or disorder, or you are just curious about this thing we call holistic wellness, I welcome you and applaud you for following your interests and your intuition. My vision of holistic wellness may be a little different from what you're used to.

I am thrilled to be able to share with you my story and what I've learned on my journey to wellness thus far. Lord knows the journey will continue for some time to come, and I look forward to sharing that as well if so guided. We are never fully healed, but we are always fully whole.

As we move through the pages of this book, I encourage you to keep a present-moment mindset. I hope none of what I share here overwhelms you. That is not my aim. I aim to meet you where you are and help you in whatever way I can. You have the power to do amazing things, and your mindset is key in that process. Take what inspires you here and run with it. Do what feels good for you at the moment and take this journey one step at a time.

For some people, that may be exploring a plant-based diet. Others may dive in headfirst as a full-on vegan. Others may try meditation or take a class. There is no wrong way to go about this. I've been working toward this lifestyle since 2015. We are all on our own journeys here, and I am blessed to be a part of your amazing journey to better health and wellness, body, mind, and spirit. I've laid it out in the order that my journey has arrived, and yours will likely look nothing like that on these pages. That's what makes it your journey.

This book is not just about eating plants or sitting in a lotus position. It's a holistic approach to finding your truly happy and healthy place in life. I will share with you all of the tools I've used and become passionate about on my journey to wellness and a whole self. I will share with you my favorite ways to have a healthy body as well as a healthy mind. Some you will resonate with and others you may not.

In 2013, I was diagnosed with Crohn's disease. That was the turning point of my life. I'd watched my mom since I was a child be allergic to everything under the sun. We were not allowed to use any scented items in our house. Imagine teenage girls with no hairspray, perfumes, nail polish, etc. Not only was she allergic to scents but a progressively increasing number of medications as well.

My mom at the time of my diagnosis had been on steroid medications for three years for Wegener's disease, and her body was starting to show signs. She was recently told that she was misdiagnosed with the Wegener's. Nonetheless, I was *not* going to take these medications, so I set out to learn all I could about how to naturally heal Crohn's disease. Of course, Crohn's disease does not go away, but it can be managed, as can many diseases in our world today. I started doing my research and soon changed my diet and found a holistic doctor.

Though it was a huge part, diet was just one component of my healing process. This is why we will explore the many other avenues of my wellness journey. These include meditation, Reiki, essential oils, crystals, and other spiritual practices. I found very quickly that if my mind was not in the right place, it sometimes did not matter what I ate. I could eat 100 percent perfectly, but if I was under too much stress or in a negative headspace, it was all over but the crying.

This may seem like a big stretch for some, but I hope you will stick with me and explore some of these avenues. They have truly been life-changing for me, and I hope they can be helpful to you as well. I ask that you proceed with an open mind and a willingness to try new things. Look beyond the things we've been told all our lives that we now take for granted as fact and truth. Explore what could be a turning point in your wellness journey. You may very well be surprised.

If there's one thing I've learned on this path, it's that food is spiritual, and spirit is food—food for our body, mind, and soul. We can feed and nourish ourselves in so many ways, and just because some may think it strange, weird, or woo-woo doesn't make it any less effective.

Throughout this journey, I have learned to appreciate more, stress less, and notice when I am doing the opposite of what feels good and works well for me. We are all different in our bodies and our minds. We each will get something different out of these pages, and what we do get is what we were meant to receive.

My goal is to help you find even one gold nugget out of my story to avoid some of the pain, some of the humiliation, and some of the fear that my journey has given me. At the same time, I hope I can help you realize that all that pain, humiliation, and fear are a blessing of some kind in your life just as mine have been for me. You may not understand that now, but someday, I hope you will.

If not for my Crohn's diagnosis, I would not be writing these pages. I would not have changed my eating and lifestyle habits, and I might just still be a stressed-out and not-so-happy person. I much prefer the person I am today, and I would love for you to find that joy as well. I hope this book opens the door to your true happiness and health for years to come. Welcome to my story.

1

THE BEGINNING

Every sunset is an opportunity to rest. Every sunrise begins with new eyes.
—Richie Norton

My mom's health was a pretty big focus in our childhood. Her allergies grew more intense and more numerous as we grew up. I remember her getting allergy testing and receiving weekly allergy shots while I was in grade school. She was allergic to dust, dander, pollen, and who knows what else. To this day, we know we cannot buy her any flowers except carnations because she's allergic to everything else. I can remember picking flowers for her and putting them in a vase out on the porch for Mother's Day.

Her food allergies were many as well: shellfish, mushrooms, coconut, and peppers. I'm not sure why I always remember shellfish but not the mushrooms and peppers. I'm forever apologizing and saying, "Mom, don't touch this—it has mushrooms in it," or "Oh shoot, I got the roasted red pepper hummus again." Sorry, Mom. Really, I am.

My dad was a carpenter but a farmer at heart. We had a small farm, and Dad was very clear throughout that the animals were not pets. The pigs were named Bacon and Sausage just to make it clear that we were not to get attached. I remember when I was twelve, my dad informed me that I was to help dress off the chickens. As he chopped the heads off and put them under a milk crate until they stopped flapping around, I was to dunk them in hot water and pull all the feathers. That day will never leave my memory. I didn't eat chicken or eggs for some time after that. Just the thought of them would turn my stomach. Looking back now, I wonder what ever brought me back to it.

The cows and the horse needed hay, so the hottest days of summer were spent haying. Of course, my mom would pass out because of sun exposure and heat exhaustion as would I at a certain point. My brother would have asthma attacks, and we would drop like flies as the day wore on. But not my sister—she was the hardcore one who got stuck with it all, all day long.

Dad would pitch the hay up onto the truck, and we would tread it in. When the truck was fully rounded up, we would ride the load up to the barn. Then we'd climb up into the hayloft. Dad would pitch it up, and we would tread until we passed out or couldn't breathe; then Dee would finish the job. Today I feel bad that she got stuck with all that.

I was never an athlete as a child either, which did not help my weight issues. It seemed every time I attempted a sport, I would get hurt or humiliated. In sixth grade, I tried out for soccer, but I couldn't run fast enough, and the ball hurt my head. That same year, I also tried out for baseball but got hit on the chin with the ball when I didn't catch it. That was the day before the school play, which I showed up to with a big black-and-blue witch chin. So I lived a sedentary childhood.

All that work provided for the milk, cream, butter, and cheese that would be made and the pounds that I would gain. I clearly remember the glass gallon jugs of milk that we would skim the cream off into a bowl, reattach the cover, and give it a shake before dinner. Then we'd whip the cream for dessert. Not to mention the homemade butter, cheese, and cottage cheese always on hand. I was a plump child, to say the least.

We had huge gardens when we were growing up as well. Family time in our house was everyone gathered around the table, snapping bushels of peas and beans, peeling carrots and apples, and making sauces, salsas, and more. Our chores included picking rocks, weeds, and potato bugs every day during the summer. We'd each be assigned three rows of weeding most days.

In today's world, we ate as clean as you could probably eat. We knew what was in our food and where it came from. There was nothing sprayed on it, injected into it, or compromised in any way. This was so unlike our food supply today, which has been tainted with herbicides and pesticides, and tampered with by scientists before it's even planted into the ground. This is not to mention the things that are injected into our meat before hitting the market with no regulation at all. Never mind the whole realm of processed foods out there with toxic ingredients that are illegal in most other countries.

Today's cows are injected with rBGH and rBST hormones to make them produce more milk. They are made to produce milk throughout their entire lives. Can you imagine nursing a child for the rest of your life?

All in all, I was raised in a pretty wholesome family atmosphere, but that didn't last forever. Once I left home, everything started to change. I continued to cook meals and eat well until I was divorced at thirty. As a single mom on a pretty strict budget, I turned to couponing, where I could get pizza rolls—ten for ten dollars down to ten for one dollar. I could get macaroni and cheese for free, as well as chips, Pop-Tarts, canned soups, and more, all of which were filled with tons of things I couldn't even read, things our bodies don't even recognize as food.

Fast-forward to 2015 when Crohn's disease made its debut. I still say couponing gave me Crohn's. I clearly remember the anxiety and humiliation every day, worrying that I would lose my job because I was never at my desk but always in the restroom. I remember as clearly as day not being able to leave the house for fear that I would not make it to the next bathroom on time. It was consuming my life. I remember my girls being embarrassed because I had to use the restroom so much anytime we went anywhere.

My diagnosis was the turning point. That was when I decided to take back my power and do something about my circumstances. I dug in and started doing the research. I learned that many people were seeing great relief from their Crohn's, UC, IBS, and on and on and on through both a vegan diet and a diet called the specific carbohydrate diet (SCD). At that time, veganism seemed a ridiculous thought. It didn't seem possible for me to take that route, so I chose the latter.

My new bible at the time became *Breaking the Vicious Cycle*, by Elaine Gottschall BA, MSc. I lived with this book by my side day in and day out. The transition was hard, but I didn't care. In a way, I've always said it was probably easier for me because I was so sick at the time that I didn't care what I had to do to feel better.

For the first week, I lived on broiled hamburgers, carrots, and chicken soup. The detox that week was crazy. The headaches were insane, and the body aches were pretty tough as well, but by the fifth day, it started to subside. My digestion had started to change. I was so happy I didn't care what I wasn't allowed to eat.

It was an adjustment though. I swear I must have gone to the grocery store every day for the first two weeks because I didn't have enough of what I needed to eat. This turned my world upside down in a very good way. By the time I hit week two, I was 100 percent committed to this program.

Once I made it through the introductory phase of the diet, I could add a few items in slowly. This diet consisted of whole foods like meat, fish, eggs, lactose-free dairy products, homemade yogurt, fresh and frozen fruits and vegetables, and beans and nuts. There was no processed or canned food allowed. No sugar, no gluten, and no messing around.

As I continued with the SCD lifestyle, my digestive issues started to improve, and I started losing the excess weight I'd collected over the years. When I was diagnosed, I was 198 pounds, which surprised me because

I'd always heard that people with Crohn's often would not be able to keep weight on whereas I couldn't get it off.

It still wasn't perfect though, and I still had occasional flares every few weeks. I remember one day in the middle of an anxiety-filled flare, taking the plunge to call and enlist the help of an old friend who had become a holistic doctor. I didn't realize it at the time, but this would be another life-changing move. He was a holistic chiropractor and used a touch-for-health modality in his practice, otherwise known as dowsing. With his help and quality supplements, I was able to progress my wellness another step further. I became a loyal patient of his until 2021 after we moved away and the two-and-a-half-hour drive didn't make sense anymore. Occasionally, when I know I'm going home, I will schedule an appointment while I'm in the area. Luckily, I'm in a much better place these days and don't need nearly as much assistance as I used to.

At this point, I realized that I had been brought down this path for a reason. I now had a passion for health and wellness, and I needed to help others who were dealing with these horrific health issues too.

This is when I enrolled at the Institute for Integrative Nutrition (IIN), another amazing turning point in my life. I realized that I could have a career doing something I was passionate about and knew about instead of continuing to follow that logical path that I'd always followed. I started my health coaching career, and I've never turned back.

I'd realized that in the accounting and tax world, I was never confident in what I was doing. When someone asked me a question, I would immediately assume I'd done something wrong. In the wellness world, I was always confident in my responses and my knowledge of the subject. This was where I belonged. It was where I thrived.

I also realized that my desire to always find a natural solution was *not* crazy and it was possible. I'd always hated taking medications over the counter or by prescription. I just never wanted anything to do with them. Now I could help people do the same.

I eventually came to realize that there were times when it didn't matter what I ate. I would still get a flare. These occasional eruptions would take me out faster than anything. I couldn't figure it out. I wasn't eating anything I wasn't supposed to, and I was still in the depths of Crohn's. I was back in that place of anxiety and fear (fear to go anywhere, fear of eating anything at all) until I realized it always happened when I was stressed out—really stressed out.

This discovery made me dig in once again. It made me start my research once again. My research brought me to meditation. I remember saying to my daughter, "I just can't figure out how to meditate." Her reply was "Mom, it's easy. Just go get the Headspace app—it's easy." So I did, and I fell in love with meditation. And another turning point surfaced.

Before I knew it I was enrolled in a certification program to become an instructor. That was truly just the beginning. My personal practice has grown immensely since then and is how I start every single day. It calms my mind and allows me to roll with life in a way that I never thought possible. We'll go deeper into meditation of all kinds in Chapter 4. Just know this is one of the main things I've been called to share with the world since those days.

It is amazing how one small decision leads to another creating that path on our journey. I know in my heart that if I'd never made that decision to download a simple app and open my mind to the concept of meditation, I would have never healed my Crohn's as well as I have, and most likely would never have written the book. I would have never in a million years signed up for a Reiki attunement class. It truly is amazing the twists and turns our life journey brings us on.

I did that Reiki class just for fun. I'd heard of it many times and had even had someone treat me with it at work once when I was having a knee issue, but I didn't really notice any difference at the time. I was intrigued, and I had been to some restorative yoga and meditation classes by this instructor, so I was already comfortable with her.

When I received my attunement, my whole world opened in a new way. This was the beginning of a new level of personal healing and progress for me. Another journey had begun, but I had no idea what an amazing turning point this would be for me at the time. I couldn't get enough. I craved everything metaphysical, creative, and weird … I've always been a little weird to a lot of people around me, so this was nothing new.

Nothing was off limits. I started my day with meditation and self-healing. I played with oracle cards, crystals, all kinds of yoga, chanting, and essential oils. I tried vegetarianism again and again. I returned to my creative roots and started drawing and painting again. Some of these things would click and others would fall away. I'd come back to some of them repeatedly, and the ones that clicked would grow from there.

At this time, I was still working my forty-plus-hour job, doing the books for a few small companies, and had also become a tax preparer while I was growing my coaching business. Looking back now, it's like I was living a double life. I just could not let go of the old one. I know now that it was all out of fear—that fear that I would fail. It was safer to work myself to death doing the thing I'd always done even though I didn't enjoy it than to step out and do what I loved full-time. It was also the money. I was enjoying all the freedom the income gave me, but was it worth all the stress and discontent it was causing?

My coaching business was all about gut health, food, and meditation. I taught cooking classes at night and did accounting by day. I coached after work, and when my clients left, I'd do the bookwork or taxes for other clients. Though I meditated all the time, I was still creating this enormous amount of stress for myself because I couldn't face my fear of failure.

In 2019, the universe decided to step in. I was laid off from my accounting job of twenty-seven years. This was no surprise. I'd seen it coming for a year prior as I watched much of my job go up the line to the upper echelon. We had come to an impasse. They needed me to expand my abilities, but I knew this was not where I wanted to expand.

So with six months of severance, I knew it was my sign that it was time to go out on my own. It was time to expand my business, or so I thought. One week later, my mother-in-law was diagnosed with kidney failure and needed dialysis three days a week. Just when you think you have things figured out, the world throws you a curveball.

I remember thinking, "Oh, *this* is why I don't have a job right now." Still determined to make my business fly, I took on the task. At the time, John was working two and a half hours away from home, and there was no one else available. Destiny, right?

One week later, I came home in tears. How the heck could I run a business if I was spending all my time waiting at the hospital for my mother-in-law, surrounded by twenty people in her situation, all in wheelchairs, and feeling helpless? It seemed impossible.

I gathered up my emotions and decided to figure it out. My new plan was to pick her up and drop her off at dialysis, go for a run, and come back and do my marketing and social media while she was at her appointments. Then I'd take her back home. I was able to turn something that would consume my entire morning into a beneficial and productive time for my health, for my business, and for her.

This worked pretty well, but as you know change is inevitable. She continued to slowly decline. There were emergencies where I needed to take her to the emergency room and sometimes to bigger hospitals farther away that could handle her issues. We'd spend whole days and weekends at the hospitals during this time. She continued to decline over the coming months until she passed in May 2019.

I'd been living my truth for the past five months, serving in a way that wasn't what I'd always imagined, but it was clearly divinely guided. My business was growing, and I was available when my family needed me. What now though? I had one month of severance left, and I needed some income. My coaching and cooking classes weren't enough. I was trying to trust that it all would fall into place, but I don't think I was doing a very good job. That trust comes hard in the beginning.

While I was planning my mother-in-law's celebration of life, my husband's uncle asked me to take a position as a manager for a local bar. Not exactly what I had in mind, but it was a part-time and managerial experience. So I took it. It would allow me to continue with my business and pay the bills at the same time.

I didn't hate this job, but again I felt like I was living a double life: hiring and managing bartenders and shopping for booze and frozen pizzas at one job and teaching people how to cook and eat organic and live healthfully at the other. Looking back, I took the safety net and was back into that double-life scenario once again.

Several months after my mother-in-law's passing, John came home and decided he had enough of the five hours of commute each day coupled with a ten- to twelve-hour workday. Now that his parents were gone, there was no desire to deal with that anymore.

We had talked about moving closer to his job for years, but it just never fell right. Now was the time. We started looking at houses and very quickly found the one we loved and put our home up for sale. One week later, it sold, and by mid-January 2020, we were in a new home in a new town.

John and I essentially switched roles at this time. I was to do the commute and he would be home at night, but I would commute up one day and back the next. We did this for three months until the country shut down, as did the bar, and once again, I was out of a job.

It was once again time to step up and make my business work. I had been doing pretty well with cooking classes and doing some organic personal chef events, and I was loving it. I was beyond excited to be really open to my skills and my passions. I felt like I was helping people lead healthier lives, but, as COVID-19's grip tightened, all this excitement was soon gone. I could no longer continue to ignore the pandemic around me and had to close my doors once again.

This also forced me to slow down and acknowledge that I was in a new home, in a new town where I knew no one at all, with no job. I was to spend all day every day with me—just me. It scared me, but I was surprised at how well I did. I immersed myself in recreating my business. I created online events, which few came to. I did live meditation classes on social media, which a few did come to, and that kept me going. I was thrilled to have anyone interested in meditation at all.

I also took this time to expand my Reiki connection and received my Reiki II and master attunements. I was like a sponge. I couldn't get enough learning and experience in the metaphysical world. By mid-2021, I'd earned my Reiki master teacher training and enrolled to earn my master's in metaphysical science.

We created a beautiful studio with a separate entrance at the house that we were so proud of. The energy in that room was amazing, but no one came. Luckily, I had been involved with essential oils, and that seemed to be doing well for the time being. I shared oils with everyone I knew for two years, but even though I loved them and was passionate about them, it was not enough.

By the end of 2021, I had to get a job. I'd tried long enough, and it just wasn't happening. I wasn't finding jobs in any field that I was passionate about, but it was time. I had to take a job. I accepted an assistant manager's job at a small family outfitter's store in the next town over. It paid the bills, and I loved the people I was working with.

My manager was sweet, and we became good friends. We were about the same age, and most of the other help was younger. I believe that job was also divinely guided. I was there to help her at a time when she could not find enough or quality help. She was there for me with encouragement and enlightenment. We supported each other in a period of tougher times but I believe we both were always grateful for all we did in those moments. I was there for five months before I found a coaching position. It broke my heart to give her the news that I was giving my two-week notice. She and I still chat back and forth, and I of course stop in to shop now and then as well. I still consider her a blessing in my life.

In mid-January 2022, I started my coaching job and that is where I remain today. I coach a metabolic reset weight loss program, which is ironic. I always said I'd never coach weight loss because I had such a hard time with that myself. Well, maybe that was the point. I have found that I truly connect with clients because of that life experience, and it is still relevant today. I still go through some of the food issues that my clients do and still must deal with them in a healthy way.

Once I was in this job, I realized that all that I'd been through had been in preparation for this moment: the time for healing and growth, the experiences, the healing that took place, and the learning how to trust that everything would always be OK and that I don't always know the best way that everything will play out in my life.

All that has led me here has given me the confidence to pursue my dreams. It has given me the confidence to step out and really pursue those dreams, write the book, get the agent, and get it published. All of this has made me realize that I am worthy of the success I dream of. Why? Because I'm living in service. My dreams are to help people feel better, thrive, and take back control of their lives and their destiny.

When people ask me the question, "If you knew you were taken care of, what would you do?" I reply, "What I am doing now but on a bigger scale. I want to share my story so that it can help others. I want to share with thousands of people at one time. I want to make a difference in how we all feel about ourselves, in our bodies, in our minds, and in spirit."

I know this journey is not done, but thus far, I can look back and truly see that every single step of the way was meant to happen and a little piece of what makes me. Each thing that I thought was a dark point in my life had its own lesson and its own piece of knowledge and growth to prepare me for where I am today and where I am going in the future.

Part of that journey includes you too. You are here right now, and I feel blessed to be part of your journey. You are part of the dream that I have dreamed. You've bought my book, which means it's been published, and that dream has been manifested and is true. Thank you.

2

SIGNS IGNORED THEN REALIZED

> The very contradictions in my life are in some way signs of God's mercy to me.
>
> —Thomas Merton

If there's anything I've learned along this journey called life, it's that we are given signs every single day. The problem is that most of us just don't see them. Don't get me wrong. I certainly don't see every single sign that is sent my way, but I do notice many more of them now than I used to.

Take for instance numerology and angel numbers. I've been aware of them for many years, and I know occasionally I would notice the synchronicities around a little prayer and the numbers showing up in my day. This was not the norm though.

I have noticed that the more I develop my spiritual connection, commit to my meditation practice, and really take care of myself, the more I notice these number signs popping up in my life. Nowadays I see these numeric signs multiple times a day. Every time I look at the clock it seems to be a significant number. Just this morning while on the treadmill, I noticed the number 2255 on my Audible time stamp on my book. The meaning?

"Divine forces are sending me a message of renewal and realignment with my spirituality."

That tells me that I'm on the right track. I've been waking up at 4:30 a.m. to do my Reiki self-healing and then getting up and going for a run on the treadmill. Not only do I feel amazed when I do that, but I'm receiving signs to keep doing what I'm doing.

Then after I got out of the shower, I looked at the clock and it was 6:44 a.m. This is a spiritual reminder from the angels that I am a person worthy of all pleasures in the world. What a great way to start the day. A pep talk from the clock. Who knew?

As I look at the clock at this very moment, I see 11:14 a.m., which encourages progressive change, renewal, and growth and asks me to share my knowledge and wisdom with others. Wow, I think I'm on the right track. I see these numbers all day every day, but there was a time when the clock was the clock and I just did not notice any of these little messages from the universe. The more I learn and the more I connect with the universe, the more I see and the less I take for granted.

These lovely little signs have made me take some time to look back on my life to see what signs I may have missed over time. The first was that time I mentioned earlier when I was twelve years old and had to help Dad dress off the chickens.

That whole experience was so overwhelming to me that my stomach turned every time I even thought about chicken or eggs. Even at twelve years old, what made beef and pork OK for me to eat? Whatever made me go back to eating chicken and eggs again anyway?

To me, this had to be a sign that the universe was sending me a message. Well, I listened for a short amount of time but eventually merged back to what everyone around me was doing—eating whatever my family was eating, doing what was normal. Then as an adult in those tough times, I resorted to cheaper versus quality foods for my family, and the story continues.

There was a point before I was diagnosed with Crohn's that my youngest daughter was sick all the time. We had her in the doctor's office every six to eight weeks. It was ridiculous. Then we connected with a great pediatrician who suggested we cut out gluten and dairy. We cut out the dairy but not the gluten because that might be hard. This did make a huge difference for her though.

Fast-forward to my diagnosis and my lifestyle change: I eliminated gluten, dairy, and any processed foods. Then as I progressed through my coaching education, I became vegetarian several times over the years. I felt better on a vegetarian diet, but I eventually went back to my old traditional and *normal* ways.

In 2021, I finally made a true commitment to my plant-based lifestyle and declared that I didn't care what anyone thought about how I ate. I didn't care if I had to make two different meals every night. I was committing to myself. The signs kept showing up throughout time, but I had not been listening. Now I was.

The longer I am plant-based, the more in tune I get with the planet, source, and my spiritual gifts. The more connected I get, the more energy I have and the more productive I am every day. Back in the day when I would run, I used to joke that I was a convenience runner. I would run until I couldn't breathe and walk until I could. I would literally not be able to run for more than three minutes at a time.

When I started running this time around after being fully plant-based for over six months, I ran twenty minutes straight on day one without stopping. My mind was blown. This is life-changing. Imagine if I never saw any of these signs.

While we're talking about signs … what about that failed marriage? When my first husband and I got together back in high school, I remember my parents not being very impressed at all. He had been in some trouble as many guys were at the time. He literally gave me his number three times, and I never called him. He did call me though. We dated through high school and moved in together once we graduated.

After finding out that he was cheating, I moved out, and my dad and a neighbor helped me do so and move back home. One week later, I moved back in. My dad was again not very impressed. He declared he'd never help me move again, understandably.

Of course, he was still not super happy that I had forgone college because I didn't want to leave the boyfriend. I'd originally planned on going to art school, then downsized to hairdressing school, and then just got a job at home so I didn't have to leave.

Hence, I went out into the world at the bottom of the ladder working in retail. While I was doing that, I earned a nutrition certification, which I loved but didn't pursue any further. I next took a job in accounting where I would spend the next twenty-seven years.

Are you starting to see a pattern? This was years prior to my marriage and my divorce, let alone my lifestyle changes.

We did have two beautiful girls once we were married, and neither one of us would trade that for those ten years of dysfunctional marriage. Those two amazing ladies astound me daily with their courage and strength and how they conduct themselves in this fear-based world.

That marriage had lessons beyond anything I could have learned in college. Though the signs were always there, so were the different paths, and I continued to choose the easier path—the less scary path. I continued that pattern for years to come as you've seen. When I received my coaching degree, I chose to keep the job and coach on the side. When I lost the job and it came down to the last scary line, I took a part-time job in the bar. When I moved and it came to the scary point again, I buckled under the pressure once more.

The signs were always there, but so were the choices and different paths. I continued to ignore those signs and took the easier path …

Once John's mom had passed and we decided to move closer to his job, I was amazed at how smoothly everything went. We only looked at houses for about three weeks. I had gone into the whole process excited and enjoying the process of looking at all the different options. The market was tough at the time. There was not much available, and when places did come on the market, they were snatched up before you could even see them.

We had found a small cabin that we were both in love with, and John was even in love more than me but was afraid it was too small. So I just put it in the universe's hands. I just trusted that what was meant to be would be. We made an offer on it and the owner turned it down, totally insulted by our offer. We counter-offered and no go. The universe had spoken.

The next weekend we'd planned on looking at more houses with our realtor, but there was one house that I'd seen on the market. I felt it was out of our price range. They were having an open house that weekend. So we planned on checking this one out before we met up with our realtor. We walked into this house where they'd already moved pretty much everything out, but they were still living there. We felt 100 percent at home.

We went home, put our current home up for sale, and put in an offer on it. One week later, our house was sold for our asking price. We closed on January 15 on the sale of our old home at noon and on the purchase of our new home at 4:30 p.m. We arrived with all our belongings at nine o'clock at night. Who would have ever imagined we could have accomplished so much in one day and have it all take place without a single hitch. That was my true realization that when you really trust that all will be OK, it really will. That was a life-changing sign for me.

My Reiki journey was very much the same. When I signed up for my initial Reiki attunement, I had no idea what I was in for. I was just curious and thought it sounded like fun, and it was. There were five of us in the group. The first part of the day was all about gaining knowledge and connection with each other. The second part of the day consisted of the actual attunement experience and our first physical experience giving Reiki to each other and our instructor.

Even though this was an amazing and almost unexplainable experience, it was nothing compared to the changes I've experienced since that day. From the moment of my attunement forward, I now see beautiful colored clouds when I close my eyes, not just the darkness I'd seen for my entire life. That was also the moment my true spiritual journey began.

My second attunement was six months later, and I was so excited to get there and find one of my best friends from high school there as well. This made the experience even more enjoyable. My master's attunement came as a great surprise. We had moved to our new home, and I wasn't even aware that the attunement was even taking place. However, I got a call from the instructor asking if I was going to join them.

In all honesty, I had no intention of going further at that point so I obviously wasn't looking. I explained that I still wasn't working and didn't really have the funds at that time, but I would release it to the universe and if the money appeared by that next day, I would join them for the class. I hung up the phone and mentioned it to John and pretty much forgot about it.

The next morning John said to me, "Are you taking the class today?" I think I looked at him like he had three heads and said, "Did I come up with $300 last night?" His response was "Candy, you started this, so you might as well finish it. Use my card." Clearly, it was meant to happen. That was my sign.

There are so many signs in life that if we were to slow down and be present in the moment, we might notice instead of letting them all pass us by. Some of these signs are just a feeling, a thought, or shall I say, a knowing. I have found that the more we pay attention to the thoughts that pop up, the things that we sometimes spontaneously blurt out because it is just there, and it happens before we know it. Those things are our intuition. That is a natural thing. That is what we were born to do. We just need to reconnect to that part of ourselves.

Back when I was a heavy drinker of wine, which was about the same time, I remember telling myself daily that I was not going to drink that day.

One thing led to another, and the next morning, I was shaming myself once again. At that time, I was using Rebecca Campbell's deck of Work Your Light oracle cards. It amazes me now to look back and see how long it took me to realize that I was receiving a sign. On those mornings when I was feeling guilty and down and beating myself up, I would always pull the Niggle card. It said, "Trust the Niggle. What is that niggling feeling trying to tell you?"[1] I clearly ignored it for about a year.

There are a lot of ways that we can do that. Giving ourselves the care we need, the respect we need, and the quiet we need to hear our own intuition is a necessity. This is important and doesn't come from just one thing or task. It comes from taking care of ourselves physically, emotionally, and spiritually. It comes from giving ourselves time to heal from broken hearts, grief, and loss. It comes from nourishing our bodies with healthy food and beverages, movement, peace and quiet, and just plain doing what we love.

The more we love ourselves, the more we can love those around us. The more we do what we love, the more energy we have for life in general. The more we do all this, the more signs and intuition we receive to guide us along the way. It doesn't matter where those signs come from, and that may be different for everyone. I see the numbers, hear the voice, pull the cards, and see all the synchronicities. Yours will likely be very different, and that's exactly the point.

Synchronicity is defined as the simultaneous occurrence of events that appear significantly related but have no discernible causal connection. When I see synchronicities in my life, I get excited. I just love these occurrences that mean something as clear as day but if we were rushing around and not paying any attention to them, would go unseen and unnoticed altogether.

John and I have a piece of property back in the town where we used to live. I've always had a feeling that we would end up back there for our retirement. We just recently had a section of it cut so that we could make a campsite, build a camp, or put up a tiny home ... We still aren't quite sure what that will look like, but when we went up to see how the job had turned out, it brought tears to my eyes. At that moment, I knew that we would retire here. We will be back, and I know this because I've come to know these feelings, my intuition, and the difference between a thought and a sign.

Thoughts pop into my head all the time, but I knew the difference the other day while talking to a client who said she'd been having more pain in her fingers and the words *uric acid* popped into my head. I pulled up her blood work and her uric acid was high. As hard as that is to explain, I knew that was a message versus just a thought. It was clearer; it was instant knowing.

Another client last week had been having a lot of heartburn. The message came to me that tomatoes were an issue. When her allergy results came in, she had a sensitivity to tomatoes and strawberries. There's always a difference between "I wonder" and "I know."

These signs can come in so many ways, not necessarily just like mine in numbers or knowledge. Maybe yours comes from a dream, something your animals may do. Have you ever thought of a friend, just to have them call on the phone at that moment?

Have you ever had technological difficulties trying to tell you something? I took a job for a large lawn care company during the COVID-19 shutdown, working as a customer service rep from home. This was one of the most stressful jobs I'd ever had. Management was watching your every move, monitoring your calls, and telling you what to say and do. The customers were all angry all the time. My husband came home one Friday evening, and I just stayed in my office quietly crying. He came in and said, "What's wrong?" I replied, "I can't stand this job. Everyone is so miserable." He replied, "Then quit!"

That night, we decided that I was already scheduled for four hours the next day and I would give my notice then. The next day when I logged on, the very first person was angry and yelling. As soon as I went to sign into his account, my computer crashed. Stressed out, I brought it all back, and my manager was telling me to save the account. I did not because this man had a legitimate complaint. I took the next call—another angry customer. Once again, as soon as I signed into his account, my computer went down. I brought it back up, and again, the manager was telling me to save the account. If this was not a sign that I did not belong here, I don't know what was. I messaged her back and said, "This is my last call. I'm logging off after this customer. I'll give you a call then."

When I talked to her, she was very nice and said that this job wasn't for everyone. I hung up and was feeling bad that I'd just quit on the spot and had never done that in my entire life. Then the manager's boss called and was really angry and informed me that the people who used their service had way too much money anyway, so they didn't really need to worry about the cost of it. I knew right there that I'd done the right thing.

We can go on living our lives as we always have, rushing around and not noticing the signs being sent out, or we can choose to slow down a little. Take the time to care for ourselves and allow the universe to guide us along the way with these little signs to make life a whole lot easier.

Have you ever found yourself suddenly emotional for no apparent reason? That was my sign when we looked at that property last month. When I saw it, I started to cry. I'd done the same thing the day we set the foundation for our old house. Some other ways that the universe may be sending you signs could be like my recurring situations with opportunities and choices for my career.

Has a song ever told you something? A scent? The weather? Words? A chill or an upset stomach? That gut feeling? A health issue? Have you ever had a plane delayed or canceled, just to realize you were much better off?

I know when I wake up in the morning with the song "You are my sunshine" in my head, it's time to go see my dad. He used to sing that to me all the time. I know the first time that happened, I didn't understand where it came from but as soon as I heard my dad's name, I knew what it was all about, and it has happened several times since.

This morning when I pulled my Isis card, as I started to shuffle the deck, I instantly had a jumper. With oracle cards, a jumper is when a card literally jumps out of the deck. I always take this as an instant message. I set the card aside and started to shuffle again. Another card jumped out of the deck. OK, then. I set it aside. Then as I shuffled again, I asked the same question I ask every day. "What do I need to know to stay on my path for the highest and best good of all today?" Then I pulled the top card.

I love the Isis oracle cards by Alana Fairchild. The card that I pulled was Abundance of Sothis. This card says, "Abundance in many forms is increasingly in flow to you. Continue your good work of building channels through which abundance can be delivered to you. Freely share your talents, love wisdom and self, and enjoy the abundance responsively flowing to you, in many forms, over and over again." This was a reminder to me to stop stressing about money and hours and to remember that I am always taken care of.[2] I know this but do tend to forget from time to time.

The first jumper card was the Eye of Horus. It reads, "The eye of Horus brings divine perception, protection, and insight. You are gifted with certain spiritual abilities, including divine sight, that are awakening and growing, now. You have much divine support and protection so that you may grow your abilities and serve others with your divine gifts. Trust your perception and know that you are divinely protected."

The second jumper was the Portal of Light, which says, "It is only this physical reality that is bound by time and space. You are a conscious being on levels beyond the physical world. You are guided to work with your healing powers beyond the confines of time and space. You will not become ungrounded through such spiritual work. You are not leaving your earthly connection behind—you are merely adding to it."

Let's see how this plays out. We already have one coach out with COVID, and I had a client email me yesterday that she was with me the day before and she was just diagnosed. All of us coaches are at this moment waiting for the results of our own COVID tests just to be on the safe side. Talk about a real time test of faith. I'm positive that my test is negative. My cards have told me so.

My test is negative as are those of the other coaches in the office. I find it amazing when I receive signs and reassurance for things that I'm not even aware of being an issue. For these cards, I was aware immediately for the first and the other seemed like general information, but now that this morning has unfolded, I can see they were much more specific than I first thought.

My favorite place to start is to take some time each day to quiet my mind. This is truly the best way to start to hear my intuition. When odd things pop into my mind for no apparent reason, I pay attention to them. I will start to notice all the coincidences and synchronicities that are here to guide me on my path. Enjoy the ride. I just love it every time I see a special number and look forward to finding its meaning. I love it when I get those meanings, imagining where it might lead. This is also part of the process. Having fun with it daily helps us enjoy each day as it progresses. It's great to receive a message of abundance coming your way, but it's also fun to spend a little time dreaming and imagining how that could show up in your life. We'll learn more about this in the manifesting chapter.

3

ADDICTION

> The only person you are destined to become
> is the person you decide to be.
> —Ralph Waldo Emerson

Addiction seems like such a shameful word, yet so many of us deal with it in some form or another. In fact, I'll bet that all of us have some sort of addictive patterns that we deal with in our lives.

My first conscious experience with addiction followed my divorce in 2002. I was not in a good mindset at that time in my life and seemed to be in a bit of a self-destructive place. I started smoking cigarettes at thirty years old. I know—who does that? Well, I did, and I continued for about five years, feeling guilty every time I lit up along the way. Actual statistics say that twenty-one million Americans have at least one addiction. Nicotine is the number one addictive substance in our country. Alcohol is number two followed by marijuana and painkillers. Then we get into the bad stuff like cocaine affecting 14 percent of Americans and heroin at 2.3 percent.

This only references substance though. There is such a thing as addiction to things, emotions, actions, etc. Over 400 million people in the world are addicted to the internet. Two hundred ten million are specifically addicted to social media. Between 27 and 30 percent of the population are workaholics. About 3 percent of the population is addicted to working out. I am not one of those.

So I smoked for five years, living with the guilt, trying to hide it from my children because I surely didn't want them to smoke. I became a professional quitter. I must have quit a hundred times in those five years. It never stuck though. I'd quit and proclaim I was done. Then I would only smoke with my friends on the weekends. Or I'd only smoke when I was drinking (bad idea, by the way). It was ridiculous how many loopholes I created to be able to smoke, be able to feel guilty, and beat myself down a little more each day.

Then one day, I decided I was tired of putting myself through this emotional roller coaster. I was done. I went out and bought all the patches I needed to fully quit so that I didn't do what I'd done in the past by being cheap and not buying the patches because they were too expensive.

Nowadays I cringe when I think of all the chemicals that must be in those patches, but I then reside with the fact that they did make me a nonsmoker. I still say that was the hardest thing I've ever done, and I swear I was a crazy woman for at least a year. I can't even imagine what people who have smoked for forty years go through.

The problem was I traded the addiction to cigarettes for an addiction to beer and food. I continued to gain weight and feel horrible but couldn't see that there was an issue. This was also the beginning of my digestive issues that would later rear their ugly head.

Once I was diagnosed with Crohn's, I realized through my research that alcohol was really bad when it came to my illness. Vodka and dry red wine were the suggestions if you had to drink. Well, I took that for the gospel and started drinking red wine. So I traded the beer for the wine. I felt this was all I had left. I couldn't smoke, I couldn't eat what I wanted, so I was going to have my wine.

It wasn't too bad to begin with, but the more I kept that mantra in my head, the more I drank. Then I figured out it was cheaper to buy more …

Yes, it's much cheaper to buy a box of wine versus four bottles. Just like our food industry—it's much cheaper to buy a burger and fries than it is to buy a salad.

This continued and got worse once we moved in 2020. I was confined to my home and had no contact with anyone but my husband. My business was failing. I had no friends and no way to meet anyone. I was falling into a state of depression, and the more I drank, the worse it got. This is when the oracle cards came in, sending me the signs that I was clearly not willing to see or hear. This went on for almost two years. I would declare, "No alcohol today," then it would be just one glass and then in the morning, the pity party and guilt trip would begin again.

I finally connected the Niggle cards to my actions and patterns on October 1, 2021. I pulled the card one more time after my little self-guilt session. The realization hit me like a brick wall, and I instantly got online and immediately discovered an AA meeting that started in five minutes. Now there's a sign.

This all happened so fast that it was almost a blur. I believe my angels were not just guiding me; they were literally pushing me in the right direction. I've had a few baby steps back but am proud to say that I am free from the grip of alcohol today and so grateful for it.

When I did join AA, I was very clear that I could not trade this addiction for food again. There was no choice here. I'd already gained thirty pounds over the pandemic, and my Crohn's was already starting to rear its ugly head. The group didn't really support this, but I stayed and received the support I could receive from them.

I consciously chose my new addiction. Yes, I chose my plant-based diet. I decided that if there was anything I could be addicted to, it had to be healthy food and a healthy lifestyle. It gave me something healthy to obsess about. I think this is key for anyone dealing with addiction of any kind. Generally, most people always replace one addiction with another without even knowing it. Once we are conscious of that, we can make the choice. We are an addictive species. We are great at forming habits, just not always good ones.

In his book *Atomic Habits*, James Clear[3] talks about how easily we form habits. The bad ones just form more easily than the good ones because we are an immediate-gratification society. When we feel tired, bored, stressed, or sad, we want to feel better, and a chocolate cupcake with chocolate frosting will do that almost immediately as we release endorphins upon the intake of sugar, whereas when we want to lose weight, stop drinking, smoking, or whatever that thing is, there is no immediate gratification because we don't have the drink, smoke, or bite of food. This is why it's harder to form good habits versus bad.

Only when we get to the misery stage of our addiction are we able to power through this scenario. This is where I was when I quit smoking *and* when I changed my diet after being diagnosed with Crohn's and when I quit drinking. Here, James Clear's habit stacking comes in handy. Stacking new habits with habits we already have in place can make this process a little more attainable. First, it refocuses our attention on the positive versus the lack of the negative. Second, it makes the new habit easier to move forward with because it almost becomes a part of the old already-established habits.

Take for example when I was drinking, I would always have a glass of wine going when I was cooking and in the kitchen. When I stopped, I just replaced the wine with a seltzer in my wine glass. I still had the wineglass going while I was cooking, but the content was much better for me. This is when I realized I really like my pretty glasses, and that was half the experience. I still do this today.

Now when I go out, I ask the waitress for some plain seltzer in a pretty glass. Most of the time, they are thrilled to oblige and think it's great. Those who don't? Well, that's their problem, not mine.

My tactic of moving to a fully plant-based diet was also helpful because I'd declared my body a temple and that I would put nothing unworthy into it. This obviously includes wine or alcohol along with any animal products or processed foods. Take note I'm certainly not saying this was easy, but I had committed myself and was bound and determined to succeed. I even had an affirmation that I still remember and use to this day. It was

"I am committed to me, my passions, goals, and my success." I use this affirmation every day. This morning I used it to get myself out of bed and again to finish my run strong.

As I repeat my affirmation throughout the day, it keeps my goals front and center as the day wears on. We all start out strong and determined in the morning, but as the day wears on, we get tired, stressed, and distracted and often we lose our resolve. Having a mantra or an affirmation to repeat throughout the day has kept me on track more times than I can count. I encourage you to create your own personal affirmation to keep moving you closer to your goals. It's done amazing things for me.

I find my affirmation especially helpful for me because it's broad enough to cover all my concerns, and in being so, it reminds me not to let other aspects of my life go as a result. I hadn't put this into action until sometime after I'd quit drinking though. I do remember one day at work after binging the night before in the candy bowl in the back room, trying to push my way through work with a migraine. I made so many mistakes that day. I shouldn't have even been at work.

I was ashamed though because I knew what had caused it: that damn candy bowl. As I walked around the store, feeling bad for myself and thinking, *What am I going to do about that candy bowl?* I remembered the words of Wayne Dyer in his book *Excuses Begone*. In that life-changing book, he explained that *everything* is in our control. "Just don't eat the candy, Candy! It's that simple" went through my mind.

When that thought crossed my mind, it was like flipping a switch. Really, Candy? Are you really going to let a bowl of candy control you? Are you really going to binge on that again tonight and deal with this again tomorrow? No, I was not, and that was the last time I did.

It's all about mindset, and once we are able to change that, we can change anything. The key is to keep it changed. I won't lie. I have fallen off the not-drinking bandwagon a couple of times, but I am relieved to say that I am now there and proud to be released from the grip of alcohol. I use this experience every day when it comes to food. Keeping my mind straight around food is no different from alcohol. I focus on my ultimate goals in life and try to remember in each moment whether this move will move me toward those goals or away. In my commitment to myself and my goals, I know if I stay focused and committed, then I will succeed in anything I put my mind to.

I also feel like I have a few secret weapons in my addiction journey. Meditation, Reiki, and my guides and angels have helped me along the way. Meditation has always been my go-to when I'm in need. I include it in my life every single day, and it keeps me focused and present. When I need a time out, I give it to myself. Who knew that would be a good thing?

Once I received my Reiki II attunement, I realized that you are never supposed to use Reiki while under the influence of anything. This was a huge help in my journey to quit drinking as well. My spiritual journey meant a huge amount to me, and I didn't want to mess it up. This realization made me much more conscious about when I would drink and how much, and I thank my Reiki guides every day for that.

I know in my heart that my daily Reiki self-healing helped me on this journey in so many ways. As I look back now, I can see myself getting more present and more conscious as time went by. This all began with my Reiki attunement. I am a true believer that people who need healing themselves should receive their attunement even if they never intend on practicing on another person. The journey is so rewarding and amazing just for personal growth and healing alone.

There are so many people in my life whom I would in a second give an attunement to help them on their journey. Reiki though is all about free will. You can't force it on anyone, but I have come to learn that the people who need it and are open will gravitate to me and it will happen in divine time.

To this day, I speak with my angels and guides before an event and ask for their help to stay committed to myself and my life goals. Just this weekend, we were at a family event where I knew everyone would be drinking. Most of them knew I wasn't drinking anymore, but there's always someone who likes to push. The morning of, I asked my guides to help me stay committed to myself and my goals while we were away. The day went off just as I wanted. As I was asked if I wanted some wine, I would have a split-second thought about it and then instantly I remembered my goals. It always feels so good to come home sober and feeling great, and even better, there's no guilt.

I am aware that my addiction is something I will always have to pay attention to. I've fallen away enough times to know that I can never let my guard down when it comes to alcohol. I always must remain conscious, present, and driven to make the right decisions at each moment. I know that this state of happiness can be taken away with just one poor decision, and I do not want to go down that road.

I have watched friends and family members fall into the grip of addiction more than once as well. Unfortunately, I've found that some cannot be reached or don't want to be reached. I know that I cannot save anyone from themselves or their addictive patterns. But the more I live for myself, my goals, and my success, the more I shine my light for others to see.

So many times, our turning point comes from somewhere totally unexpected or even unexplained. It comes from someone else shining their light, being their true self, and living their best life. We don't have to save anyone; they need to save themselves. All we can do is save ourselves.

When coaching, one of my biggest things is to get people to take care of themselves. Self-care is not greed; it's self-preservation. The more we take care of ourselves, the more we shine our light out to the rest of the world and that's all we have to do. Isn't that a crazy thought that all I have to do is take care of myself? Yes! *And* it removes so much pressure, drama, and anxiety. I don't have to worry about anyone else, just me! What a concept. It makes everything so much more manageable.

When you stop and think of it, maybe that's how we got here in the first place. In Alcoholics Anonymous, they ask, "What in your life was unmanageable?" Maybe it was trying to manage everyone else instead of focusing on our own needs and letting the rest all fall into place.

If there's one thing I've learned on my journey to sobriety, it's that the job is never complete. This is a lifetime journey for me. I have come to realize that I will always have to be conscious and aware in each moment because it takes the slightest misstep for me to be on the other end of sobriety.

I have decided that it is manageable though. It has given me license to let go of things that are less important in my life to remain healthy, happy, and inspired to share my journey with the world. By letting go of those things that I used to think were important, I can manage what is.

Self-care is *the* most important thing. I don't care what anyone says about that. Those who call self-care greedy or selfish are just neglecting themselves as well as those around them. When we love and care for ourselves, we are more able to love and care for those we love and care for.

We recharge and reinspire ourselves to share all that we have to offer. Isn't that what this world is all about? Sharing each one of our pieces of individuality? What makes us each different from the other? That which makes us truly ourselves in our own right?

As scary a statement as it is to make, I pledge to keep my sobriety. I continue to stay sober and present a high vibration so that I can truly do my part in making this world a better place. I can't do that in a drunken stupor.

Unfortunately, our society touts alcohol as part of our culture and a sign of success. It is sad to me that every ad you see on television shows people with a beer, drink, or glass of wine in hand. This used to be a real trigger for me. No joke, my mouth would water when I saw a glass of wine on television, and instantly, I would want one. For those just starting their sobriety journey, this is a tough thing to face every day.

According to https://pubs.niaaa.nih.gov, alcohol commercials make up *1.5 percent of all advertisements on primetime television and 7.0 percent of all advertisements in sports programming.*[4]

Not only is it plastered all over our ads but throughout the shows, movies, and other programming we watch every day. This has created a misleading idea that it is OK to take part regularly.

It often starts out kicking off the weekend, then it becomes the weekend or may become a nightly glass of wine or beer or drink after a long day. Then it progresses from a drink a night to two or three and then just too much once in a while. When it progressed to a bottle-a-day habit, it was when I realized I had an issue and it wasn't just to relax.

I was not dealing with my emotions. I was drowning them out because I didn't want to deal with them. I was raised to be tough and not be a baby, so dealing with my emotions wasn't a choice. Or was it?

I eventually found out it was. I eventually realized I *always* have a choice. Whether it was comfortable or not was a different matter, but one way or another, it had to be dealt with. I had to deal with what wasn't manageable in my life.

What I thought wasn't manageable was that I was in a pandemic and I had no job, no friends, no life. What I really found in the end was the emotions I'd buried years ago from a failed marriage, lifelong weight issues, and childhood traumas were what was not manageable.

I couldn't bury them anymore. They were leaching out of my pores with the stench of alcohol, and I had to deal with it one way or another. The pandemic wasn't the cause; it was part of the solution. I believe the pandemic provided this for many of us—time to sit with ourselves and our feelings and finally feel them and deal with them instead of drowning them day after day, week after week, and month after month.

When you are truly alone and at your lowest, you have no choice but to see the truth about yourself. Thank God for that. This is why people bless the day they hit rock bottom—because it was a turning point. The realization that I didn't want to live this way anymore was pivotal for me, and I truly am grateful for the two years it took me to get there as well as the long climb back.

That climb has made today so much more gratifying and blissful. In that process, I found blessings, abilities, and gifts I never knew I had. I found strength and courage instead of weakness and fear.

When we remove the veil, we can expose the beauty within us and let it all shine for the world to see. Addiction is the veil that we think no one sees. But it doesn't matter what anyone else sees. It matters what we see, believe, and love about ourselves. We, ourselves are what matters the most, and if we all believed that from a non-ego place, then this world could be an amazing and loving beautiful place.

My addiction journey started a long time before I realized I had an addiction issue. It had been growing a long time before I had an inkling that it was there. I ignored the signs for a long time. Those signs were there early and got louder and louder the longer I did not listen. Soon they were in my face and so obvious that I could no longer ignore them. If you are receiving the signs, don't ignore them any longer. Reach out for help, there are so many organizations that can help you escape the clutches of addiction.

I've spent a lot of time in what they call the gray area of drinking, during my recovery, relapse, and repeat stages—that area where I was neither an occasional drinker nor an alcoholic. But then it always led back to too much. It wasn't until I really realized and faced the fact that this habit was not helping any of my pillars of wellness, physically, emotionally, or spiritually.

Alcohol does nothing good for us. I know we have been marketed a totally different story. We're sold the idea that it's sexy, healthy, normal, and earned. Yes, you know what I'm talking about. Friday night when you're doing your groceries and you think, "I've worked hard this week. I deserve some wine," never having intentions of drinking the whole bottle. Yet it happens. Even if it doesn't, two or three glasses disrupt your sleep, give you a headache, and result in inflammation in the body.

The body metabolizes alcohol into acetaldehyde; this damages DNA and keeps it from doing its job of repairing damage. Once DNA is damaged, a cell can grow out of control into cancerous cells.

Research finds even light drinking increases the risk of high blood pressure and heart disease. This risk increases dramatically as intake increases. The American Cancer Society attributes alcohol to 75,000 cases of cancer a year. They point it out as a direct cause of head and neck, esophageal, liver, breast, and colorectal cancers.

We all know our liver is affected by excess alcohol, but while the liver is processing alcohol, it stops releasing glucose. This results in low blood sugar levels, which happen at a much faster rate than would normally.

It's clear that alcohol is just not good for us in any way. That made me realize that I work so hard in every other area of my life to be healthy, vibrant, and energized, so why would I put this poison into my body?

It wasn't easy, but it was worth every single struggle, tear, and hurdle when I could see the light on the other end of that bottle and when I saw how amazing life could be with clarity and a heart filled with love for myself again. I am worth it and so are you if you're struggling with it.

4

MEDITATION, TRULY LIFE-CHANGING FOR ME

> Meditation isn't just something we do to make ourselves more peaceful and to take some of the stress out of our lives. We do it because it's the only direct experience we can have of knowing God, whatever that means for you.
>
> —Wayne Dyer

Though I have many passions, meditation is one of my true passions in life, so much so that I am grateful for the low points in life that led me to this path. With my Crohn's diagnosis came an immense amount of stress and anxiety. I distinctly remember fearing the loss of my job because I was never at my desk. The image of the anxiety of even the thought of leaving the house is still clear as a bell in my mind.

These are the things that had me grasping at straws for solutions. I remember the desperation to try anything that had the smallest chance of making a difference. The thing I didn't realize was that I was in a vicious cycle. Even after changing my diet and seeing some improvement, that stress and anxiety would spark flares that I could not figure out and could not manage.

The first time I tried meditation, I knew this was something big. Even though I didn't see some big miraculous change, I knew deep in my soul that this was the answer I was looking for. Little did I know it would become part of my life's path, the thing I most needed to share with the world.

Meditation was one of the first areas where I really got serious about my self-care. Just ten to fifteen minutes a day made such a big difference in how I felt every day that I was hooked. I couldn't believe such a simple thing could calm my mind as well as my body. I became less stressed, and it was that extra edge my body needed to start to really heal.

The more I did it, the more I loved it, and before I knew it, I had enrolled in a teacher certification program. I couldn't get enough of it. Once I started my studies though, I found myself very judgmental of my ability to quiet the mind. Yes, me too. This is where we all go when we begin. My instructor finally got it drilled into my head to not judge the process. There is a reason why it is called practice. We are practicing.

We are human, and our minds are not meant to shut off. They also aren't meant to be in high gear 100 percent of the time. The key is to quiet the mind, not shut it off. Thoughts will continue to come, but with practice, we can slow that constant chatter down and just observe the thoughts as they pass by.

When I was immersed in my studies, I would meditate for an hour a day no matter what my state of mind was or how well the process went. I would force myself to sit there for an entire hour, trying to quiet my monkey mind.

Then I realized that forcing the issue just brings on other thoughts of frustration and doesn't really help with relaxation at all. In fact, it is much more effective to take ten minutes a day to meditate every day than it is to meditate for sixty minutes once per week. So if you feel like you don't have the patience to sit for a long meditation, then no worries. You're better off starting with five or ten minutes every day anyway.

There are many misconceptions about meditation, and even though its rich history goes back thousands of years, there is still a stigma around it today. Meditation is not hypnotism, a cult thing, a way to escape from life, for hippies and weirdos. It's not a religion, though many religions, in fact, most religions also have their own history in meditation. Jesus meditated on the mountain; Buddhism came out of meditation. Meditation is coming to a peaceful place of contemplation and allowing the noise to still for a bit.

I remember my beloved and very passionate Christian uncle asking me once if I was comfortable enough in my own religion to be dabbling in others. I explained that meditation was just quieting the mind and focusing on something intently like breathing. It is a practice of quieting the mind, not a religion. I explained it can be used in any religion, but it is not a religion.

In the very beginning, I started with the Headspace app, and I loved the little guy with the Aussie accent. It just made me happy. Later, I found the Insight Timer app and used it forever. Today I am an instructor on Insight Timer as well as a regular user. Insight Timer has so much to offer from meditations to yoga and life workshops. The app is free with the option to a premium plan if you wish. Check it out and see what you think at www.insighttimer.com or you can check out my page at https://insighttimer.com/candyspassion. It truly is my passion and I enjoy creating, channeling, and sharing new meditations as they come to me.

I really believe there is a huge need for meditation in everyone's life. It can be used for so many things and much more than just quieting the mind. I use it to figure out decisions that I'm having a problem with and more like reducing stress, self-love, self-empowerment, reflection, weight loss, manifesting, and sleep.

There is so much research out there connecting the benefits of meditation on anxiety and depression, weight loss, meeting goals and achievements, and more. Transcendental meditation has provided enormous success to veterans dealing with PTSD and more. Ho'oponopono meditation has been credited with closing down a high-security prison for the criminally insane in Hawaii with the help of therapist Dr. Len. There are many kinds of meditation such as spiritual, focused, movement, mantra, transcendental, loving-kindness, visualization, and mindfulness, to mention a few.

I am a mindfulness meditation instructor who, for the most part, focuses on the breath. I love this because it makes it possible to meditate anywhere. You always have your breath with you. I am also an instructor on Ho'oponopono, which can also be done anywhere but works on a bit of a different theory than most other genres.

Not only is there a huge need for meditation individually, it is so important worldwide today. Take the example of the Maharishi effect. According to https://maharishi-india.org/maharishi-effect, in 1975, Maharishi inaugurated the dawn of a new era, proclaiming that 'through the window of science we see the dawn of the Age of Enlightenment.

Scientific research has found that in cities and towns all over the world where as little as 1 percent of the population practices the transcendental meditation (TM) technique, the trend of rising crime is reversed, and order and harmony are increased. The scientists named this the Maharishi effect the same as his namesake.

The Maharishi effect sets the principle that individual consciousness affects collective consciousness. Almost fifty scientific studies over the past twenty-five years confirm the effect and wide-ranging benefits to the nation produced by the Maharishi effect. These studies have used rigorous research methods and evaluation procedures available.

The influence of coherence created by the Maharishi effect can be measured both nationally and internationally. Increased coherence within a nation expresses itself in better harmony and well-being as a nation. This harmony also creates an influence that extends beyond the national borders, improving international relations and reducing conflicts. In reality, we really can create peace in our world.

I belong to an empath group where we get together via Zoom on a weekly basis to help support each other on our empathic journeys. We also do a group meditation at 9:00 a.m. on Sundays and 9:00 p.m. on Wednesdays. We all do our own meditation in the comfort of our own homes but at the same timing as to maximize our loving energy.

Another amazing tool that helped me move past my first marriage and divorce was the loving-kindness meditation. This practice is amazing when you have people you need to forgive and bring true peace back into your life. I will include this at the end of the chapter for your use.

The loving-kindness meditation guides you to love everyone no matter what. This is a great tool when dealing with resentment and anger toward someone in your life. I found it very helpful and would recommend it to anyone having a hard time forgiving someone. Remember forgiveness is to free you, not them.

I especially love Louise Hay's response to meditation: "Every time you meditate, every time you do visualization for healing, every time you say something for healing the whole planet, you are connecting with like-minded people all over the planet who are doing the same thing." So very true. God rest her soul.

Loving-Kindness Meditation

Close your eyes. Sit comfortably with your feet flat on the floor and your spine straight. Relax your whole body. Keep your eyes closed throughout the whole visualization and bring your awareness inward. Without straining or concentrating, just relax. Take a deep breath in. And breathe out.

Receiving Loving-Kindness

Keeping your eyes closed, think of a person close to you who loves you very much. Imagine that person standing in front of you, sending you their love. That person is sending you wishes for your safety, well-being, and happiness. Feel the warm wishes and love coming from them to you. Now imagine that you are surrounded by all the people who love you and have loved you. Picture all your friends and loved ones around you. They are standing, sending you wishes for your happiness, well-being, and health. Bask in the warm wishes and love coming from all sides. You are filled and overflowing with warmth and love.

Sending Loving-Kindness to Loved Ones

Picture a person that you love. Begin to send the love that you feel back to that person. You and this person are similar. Just like you, this person wishes to be happy and have a good life. Send all your love and warm wishes to that person. Repeat the following phrase silently: Just as I wish, may you live with ease, may you be happy, may you be safe and healthy (repeat three times).

Sending Loving-Kindness to Neutral People

Now think of an acquaintance, someone you don't know very well and toward whom you do not have any particular feelings. You and this person are alike in your wish to have a good life. Like you, this person wishes to experience joy and happiness in his or her life. Send all your wishes for well-being to that person, repeating the following phrase silently: Just as I wish to, may you live with ease, may you be happy, may you be safe and healthy (repeat three times).

Sending Loving-Kindness to Enemies

Now think of someone that you may not get along with. Call the difficult person to mind and be honest about what you feel. There may well be feelings of discomfort. Notice any tendency you may have to think badly of that person, or to deepen the conflict you have with them and let go of these tendencies. Instead, wish them well, repeating the following phrase silently: Just as I wish, may you live with ease, may you be happy, may you be safe and healthy (repeat three times).

Sending Loving-Kindness to All Living Beings

Now, expand your awareness and picture the whole world in front of you as a little ball. Send warm wishes to all living beings on the earth who, like you, want to be happy: Just as I wish too, may you live with ease, may you be happy, and may you be safe and healthy (repeat three times).

Take a deep breath in. And breathe out. Take another deep breath in and let it go. Notice the state of your mind and how you feel after this meditation.

When you're ready, you may open your eyes.

https://www.nantien.org.au/[5]

Here are a few meditations that I created. I hope you enjoy them and find them helpful in even the smallest way. You can find the soundtrack at www.candyholmesfoster.com/bonus.

Meditation to Anchor, Align, and Arise

Every now and then, we just need to stop the chaos around us and take some time to get grounded and realigned to rise up. So today we are going to anchor, align, and arise. There is so much to be said about taking the time out for yourself, to get grounded, to collect your thoughts and energy in order to move forward. Congratulations on taking care of yourself.

Find a comfortable position with a nice straight spine. You can be sitting, lying down, or even standing if you'd like. Take a deep breath in and fully fill the lungs, and release. Let it all go, all the stuff that's got you feeling out of control, out of alignment, and scattered. Just let it go with that exhalation.

Take another deep breath in and fill those lungs. Blow that breath back out through the mouth. Let it go.

Breathe in deeply one more time and hold it at the top of your breath for just a moment. Now slowly let it all go out through the mouth.

Come back to a softer, gentler, more natural breath. Fall into the rhythm of the breath and follow it with your mind, letting everything else go. Follow that breath in and out as your chest rises and falls. Follow it.

Notice the effects of gravity on your body, where you are in your physical space. Feel the surface beneath you. Make that connection between your feet and the floor, your bum and the chair, your body and the bed, the couch, or the floor. Whatever it is, recognize the security that whatever is beneath you provides—the safety, the stability. Feel it.

Imagine roots growing down through that surface toward the earth. When it reaches the earth, it burrows down, down, down until it reaches the pure center of the planet. You are rooted in Mother Earth. Feel the security this brings you. Sit with this feeling of safety for a moment.

As you sit in this secure space, feel your nervous system start to settle, calm and quiet. Feel that frantic edge on your emotions soften and start to let go. Continue to breathe slowly and steadily.

When you notice thoughts pushing their way in, just acknowledge them and let them pass by with the next breath. Just like the breath, allow it to come and go with no judgment. Become the observer and just watch it all pass by.

As you settle into this calmer state, remind yourself that all is well. Start to align with this thought. All is well. All is well. All is well.

Sometimes we get so wrapped up in the intensity of our lives that we forget that we are always taken care of and that all is truly well. Align with the feeling and the energy of this though. All is well.

Allow your physical body to align with this energy. Allow your body to slow down and start to align with your mental body. Allow your emotional body to fall into this alignment too. Feel them synchronize and start to flow with the breath. Feel the calm settle over you.

Sit with these feelings for a bit and just breathe.

Now that you are just the observer, you can bring back to your consciousness the situation that had you so out of alignment.

Now you can take an outside look at the situation. Observe and imagine how to approach it differently. How can the problem be solved? Is there a different angle to look at it from? Is it even as important as you once thought it was?

Sit with this for a bit and just ponder, unattached—without judgment.

Now whether you've found a solution or not, just let this all pass by just like those thoughts and the breath. Allow yourself the space to let this go and rise above it.

Feel a sense of release, feel a weight lifted, and allow yourself to rise above it. Let the situation go and feel the gratitude that you were able to release yourself from its grip. Arise.

Feel your energy restored, your spirit refreshed, and your vibration rising up. Arise, arise, arise.

It's now time to come back to your physical space. Recognize all that is around you. Start to wiggle your fingers and toes and come back when you're ready.

Thank you for joining me today, and I hope this time has brought you a sense of renewed clarity and balanced energy. May you have peace.

Namaste.

Meditation to Connect with Nature

Our modern-day lifestyles often don't allow for as much time in nature as we truly need. Getting out and being one with nature keeps us grounded, recharged, and present. I love to do this meditation outside sitting on the ground or maybe even leaning up against a favorite tree. I've done it on a rock by a stream or on the dock on the lake.

Of course, you can also do it inside in your favorite chair and just use your imagination. Wherever works best and inspires you the most is the perfect place to start.

So let's find that place where you can settle in. Find a nice straight spine to allow for a good flow of energy and let's take a deep breath in and release.

Take another deep breath in, filling the lungs and the stomach. Then let it all go out through the mouth.

Let's take one more deep breath in and release fully.

Start to fall into a softer, gentler, more natural breath. Continue to follow that breath in and out, in through the nose, throat, lungs, stomach, and back out the stomach, lungs, throat, and nose. Slow and steady. Soft and gentle.

Start to notice the effects of gravity on your body. Feel your heaviness on the surface beneath you. Really notice that connection. If you're not in nature, imagine the surface beneath being the grass, sand, a rock. Whatever and wherever you would love to be in nature.

Allow roots to grow down into the earth like the tree beside you, growing deeper and deeper until they reach the center of the planet. Feel the security that comes with this connection. Allow this security to soothe your nerves and calm your mind.

Feel the energy coming back to your body with this connection, recharging your body, mind, and spirit.

As you continue to breathe in your mind's eye, notice all of nature around you. What surrounds you in this place? Is it water, trees, or fields?

What does the air feel like? Is the temperature warm or cool? Take it all in and allow it all to calm your senses.

Is there an aroma in the air? What do you smell? How does that make you feel?

If you notice tension rising, just take a deeper breath and let it go on the exhalation. Allow the release.

What is happening around you? Just observe the leaves, water, birds, and whatever is around to pass by and do their thing. You can just sit and watch and enjoy. Soak in all the miracles of nature.

Breathe in the fresh air and feel it refresh you from the inside out. Let it fill you up. Allow yourself to truly let go of the outside world for a while and just enjoy this place of peace and wonder.

If thoughts start to invade this precious space, acknowledge them and just let them pass by like the leaves or water in the stream and come back to your place of peacefulness.

Notice all you are grateful for at this moment. Right here and now, what feels good? What is making you happy right now? Bring those things to mind and start to roll with all the other things that come up, all the blessings in your life.

Feel that gratitude and let that feeling grow and multiply. Let it take over your thoughts. Feel your heart filled with joy, peace, and gratitude. Feel it, love it, embrace it.

Take one last look around you and notice anything you have not seen before. See the beauty that surrounds you, the beauty that surrounds us every day.

Make a commitment to come back here every day, reconnect with nature, and find your peace again. You are worth it.

Start to come back to the here and now, your physical space, acknowledge your surroundings, and start to wiggle your fingers and toes. Let's take a deep breath in … and release.

I am so blessed to have you join me today. Thank you and may your day be filled with the joy of nature,

Namaste.

Self-Empowerment Meditation

My struggles and experiences in life are what drive me to do what I do. On my journey, I have found that 90 percent of the time, no matter what we're dealing with, mindset is key. Mindset plays such a huge part in our success or failure at everything we do.

How do we get our head in the game and keep it there though? That is precisely why I created this meditation. To help us all keep our heads in the game, inspired, motivated, and self-empowered. Are you ready? Then let's do this.

Please find yourself a comfortable space where you can relax but have a nice straight spine. Our spine is like a train track for our energy. So the straighter it is, the better the energy flows.

Let's take a deep breath in through the nose. And let it all go out through the mouth.

Take another deep breath in and release fully.

One more deep breath in and let it all go.

Come back to a softer, gentler, more natural breath and just settle into it. Allow it to nurture and calm the body and the mind. Let the breath help you settle and relax.

Bring to mind something you may have been struggling with lately but as an observer only, judgment-free and with no attachment.

From this place, we can more clearly analyze the situation. Ask yourself these questions.

> What has not been working?
> What needs to be done?
> Why haven't I done it?
> Am I making excuses? Why?
> Am I afraid? Why?
> What am I afraid of?
> What is my next best move?
> When will I do it?
> Am I procrastinating? Why?
> Now when will I do it?

Facing our fears and getting out of our own way is the first step toward accomplishing our goals. Once we face our fears, we can move forward.

Now that you know what you need to do and when you'll do it, visualize it. Yes, right now.

Recite this affirmation to yourself right now: "I am committed to me, my passions, my goals, and my success."

Now bring your mind to that moment—that moment when you are going to move forward and take that next step.

Recite again, "I am committed to me, my passions, my goals, and my success."

Visualize being there ready to do it.

Again say, "I am committed to me, my passions, my goals, and my success."

Visualize actually taking that step and following through. How does this feel? You're doing it. Feel it and know what it feels like. Keep visualizing it as long as you need to be successful.

I am committed to me, my passions, my goals, and my success.
I am committed to me, my passions, my goals, and my success.
I am committed to me, my passions, my goals, and my success.

You are on your way to success. Be the success you want to be, meet the goals you want to meet, and live the passions you want to live. You have the power to do anything you can dream possible, so step out of your shadow and shine for the world to see.

Start to come back to the breath, come back to the here and now and your physical space. Deepen your breath and open your eyes when you're ready.

I suggest you come back to this meditation daily as long as you need to. Sometimes your goals may change, but the process is the same. Keep your head in the game and empower yourself.

Thank you for joining me today and enjoy your newly accomplished success.

Namaste.

Self-Reflection Meditation

This can be a great practice coming into a new moon as a way of letting go of the old and to welcome in the new. Self-reflection is key in moving forward on our paths no matter what that path is. By reflecting on what we've done or not done, we can learn and choose accordingly in the future.

So let's get settled in and let's find a comfortable place where we can spend a little time quietly. Let's find a nice straight spine and let's begin.

Please take a deep breath in and release, emptying your lungs fully.

Take another deep breath in. Follow the breath as it fills your lungs and your belly expands. And release fully.

Take one more deep breath in and hold for a moment at the top of the breath and then slowly and softly release the breath.

Come back to a softer, gentler, and more natural breath, and allow each inhalation to bring in new, fresh energy and each exhalation to take away anything that does not serve you at this time.

Let each breath cycle relax your body and your mind a little more.

We are now in the present moment as we follow the breath.

Let's take a trip back in time. Go back to the beginning of this month and observe the goals that you had set for this month, with true detachment as you just observe.

What were your goals for this month?

Did you attain these goals or make progress toward them? Observe each goal and its current state, free from emotional attachment.

Were some goals not attained?

What might have stood in the way of this? Is there something you might do differently?

Just sit with it for a bit with an accepting mindset, a mindset flowing with life and all its peaks and valleys.

Sometimes we push too hard to attain our goals and others we don't push enough. Being able to reflect on all those actions and allow yourself to flow with them can sometimes bring us to that place of success with more enjoyment and less stress.

Now reflect on how you may have responded in the moments when things didn't quite go as planned. Reimagine yourself handling it differently, flowing with the situation with ease and grace.

Remind yourself that when things don't work out as we planned, that usually means there's something better ahead, something greater in store for you.

Now just surrender to this thought. Feel gratitude that something better is in store and maybe you just need to reassess the situation for other options and opportunities.

Sometimes as we reflect, we even find that the goal is no longer valid or no longer fits with our current path, and that is fine too. Again, feel gratitude for this discovery.

Flow with gratitude for a little bit. Let it grow into more and more things you are grateful for as you reflect. Enjoy noticing the blessings.

Now take a moment to reimagine the coming month. Imagine everything happening in perfect order, in perfect flow, in perfect timing, and better than you ever imagined.

Dream and imagine it all coming together perfectly.

Start to come back to your physical space. Come back to this room and your placement in the room. Take a deep breath in and release.

Start to wiggle your fingers and toes and come back when you're ready.

Meditation to Raise your Vibration

We all have those days when we wake up just feeling blah. This morning was one of those days for me. It's a Monday and we didn't get home until late last night, so we didn't have much time to unwind before bed and that is usually a recipe for the blahs the next day. It was, but I have learned to never accept that into my life.

Raising my vibration on those days is imperative to me. The more time I spend in high vibration, the more I don't like the times I'm not. So if you're having a blah day, you're in the right place. Let's raise it up.

Find yourself a quiet space that feels good to you. Settle into a comfortable position where you can sit for a while and have a nice straight spine.

And take a deep cleansing breath in ... and out.

Take another deep replenishing breath in ... and let it all go out through the mouth.

One more time, let's take a deep breath in ... and release it fully out through the mouth.

Come back to a softer, gentler, and more natural breath, and allow yourself to relax into it. Allow each breath to soothe your nervous system, calm your mind, and relax your body with each exhalation.

Come to the place in this present moment and allow yourself to step back and just observe. Take a moment to check your mood. How do you feel right now? Make note of that feeling without judgment. Just observe what it is.

Continue to slowly and steadily follow each breath in and out, in and out. In ... and out.

Feel the tension leave your body. Feel it leave your chest with each exhalation, softening the body and relaxing the mind a little more with each cycle.

No matter what lower vibrations you may be feeling in this moment, allow the breath to take a little more of it away with the exhale. Allow the inhale to bring in the newer, replenished, and inspired higher vibrations. Feel your body and mind filling up with this positive energy twofold.

Imagine every time you exhale, you lose one drop of negatively charged water, and with every inhalation, you take in two positive ones. Feel your well filling up more and more with each breath with bright, clear, and regenerative water.

This water will hydrate your body, mind, and spirit as it continues to cleanse you of all that does not serve you right now. Take some time now to fill yourself up more and more with each breath.

As your vessel fills up more and more, feel the difference in your mood. Is it feeling more inspired? More present, content, even happy? Can you feel gratitude at this moment?

Allow these feelings to overflow and spill out for the rest of the world. Share your contentment and joy with the world. Share how it feels to be happy so the next person can feel it and share it too.

Allow these feelings to inspire you further. What do you want to do today? What do you want to accomplish? How do you want to play and dance with life?

Declare it now and do it today. Flow with your higher vibration and feel it grow within you even more. Allow happiness to build, the contentment to grow and the joy to blossom into the bright beautiful flower that you are meant to be, with the biggest, brightest blossoms you've ever seen.

Share this feeling with the world and allow others to take on your energy and joy. Inspire others to do the same and rise into this great community of happiness and beauty.

Sit with this higher vibration for a moment and just enjoy how it flows through you.

In your mind's eye, take a snapshot of this moment in time. Save this in the back of your mind for any time you may be feeling low. Remember you always have the ability to raise yourself up from any lower vibration. You have that power.

Start to deepen your breath. Take one more deep breath in and release.

Start to come back to the here and now. Start to notice your surroundings and fully come back when you're ready.

Thank you so much for joining me today. I am honored to share this time with you and to be able to help elevate your day.

With joy and love

Namaste.

Mindfulness Practice for a Restful Night's Sleep

Sleep is such a huge contributor to our overall wellness, so it's important to create a good practice with an evening routine that starts to bring your energy levels down as you approach your time to retire for the evening.

I am honored to be part of that practice this evening, and I hope this meditation can assist in your sleep journey every evening. If you drift off before the meditation is complete, no worries at all just allow your sleep to settle in. I always suggest getting ready for and getting comfortable in your bed so that when you drift off, you can stay in slumber.

Please settle into bed and allow your whole body to relax. Observe the true comfort of your bed. Enjoy the feeling of your covers embracing every curve of your body, making you cozy and warm. Feel the comfort of your pillow forming to the curve of your neck with full supportive comfort.

Take a deep breath through your nose, allow it to fill your lungs, and let your belly expand. As you release that breath out through the mouth, let the belly deflate as you release. Feel how the covers move softly with the movement of your body.

Take another deep breath in and allow the belly to expand and release fully through the mouth once more.

Let's take one more deep breath, fully filling the lungs and belly, and then let it all go out through the mouth.

Settle into a softer, gentler, more natural breath, following it in and out with your mind, letting go of any thoughts lingering from the day. As you breathe, let those thoughts just drift by. As they do, release any attachment to them. Just observe them floating away.

If you're already anticipating tasks and things tomorrow, let's take a moment to imagine your day unfolding from the time you awake throughout the day and bringing you right back here. Imagine every task going smoothly, every conversation a pleasure, every event turning out just as you imagined or better.

As you feel the contentment of tomorrow unfolding in its perfection, come back to the breath. Notice how relaxed you are. You've released your weight to the bed. Your muscles are relaxed. The tension in your chest is gone, and you feel truly relaxed.

Continue to follow the breath, and it starts to drift away as you drift off to sleep and peaceful dreams.

Sleep well, my dear.

Namaste.

Step into Your Dreams

This meditation came to me as I was listening to the 2023 Hay House "You can heal your life" summit. Rebecca Campbell was speaking on living a soul-led life. Rebecca is one of my favorite authors and spiritual sisters and she has brought me so much guidance on this journey. This week I am on vacation and not going anywhere but just burning time before I lose it. I'd spent some time wondering what I would do with myself for an entire week but soon created a long list of things I'd been meaning to do. Write, create meditations, create a book proposal, work out daily, and continue with my studies. You get the idea.

While listening to Rebecca, I realized that I have fallen back into old habits of resistance, resisting the things that I need to do to claim my dreams. That book won't write itself and those meditations won't record themselves. If I don't write and record, then I can't share what I want to share with the world. I'm assuming you all do this too. So let's leave that all behind and step into our dreams.

Find a comfortable position and settle in. Take a deep breath in and release. In fully and out fully. One more time, in with a deep full breath and out with all of that resistance. Close your eyes and start to breathe softer, more naturally. Allow that breath to calm you.

Let each exhalation take away a little more of the resistance you're holding on to. No matter what this resistance resides around, let it go.

Often, we are in a subconscious state of fear. Fear of failure or even fear of success. Let it go. Breathe it out. Let it go ...

Follow that breath in through your body ... and out through your body. Let go of all that fear and procrastination.

Bring your mind to your dreams. What is it you want to do, be, and share with the world? What is that big thing you want to bring to your life and the world? Bring it front and center.

Allow it to grow and evolve.

Feel it, hear it, smell it, and taste it.

Now what is one tiny step you can take in that direction? What is holding you back? What are you afraid of? Why are you resisting? Feel that fear, that resistance, and let it go on your next exhalation. Breathe in new energy and purpose. Breathe out the fear and blocks.

Visualize doing that thing you're shying away from. Move forward, see it. Know that this is the only way to get there—one step in front of the other. Take one step, then another, then another, over and over again.

Can you feel the momentum? Feel your soul start to rejoice and sing. This is where you will realize your dreams. This is where you become the success you dream of. This is where it all begins.

It is time to come back to the here and now. Recognize the space you are in, take a deep breath in, and release. Open your eyes when you're ready.

Now I would recommend getting a drink of water and deciding what is your next step and taking it. Step into your dreams now.

Namaste.

You can find these recordings on my website at www.candyholmesfoster.com/bonus.

5

REIKI BROUGHT ME PEACE

> Reiki is love,
> Love is wholeness,
> Wholeness is balance,
> Balance is well-being,
> Well-being is freedom from disease.
>
> —Mikao Usui

May I just say that when I entered the world of Reiki, I had no idea what I was in for. I honestly thought it would just be a fun weekend meeting some new people and exploring something new and different. That was certainly an understatement, to say the least.

I was trained in the Usui tradition of Reiki. There are about twenty-five different types of Reiki, which are offshoots from the original Reiki imparted by Dr. Usui. Mikao Usui was the founder of Reiki, which is practiced all over the world. Hawayo Takata, a Japanese woman, spread the teachings of Reiki to the West after Dr. Usui's passing.

Reiki is a Japanese energy healing technique that involves the transfer of energy or qi through a practitioner's palms, usually through direct touch or the laying of hands. In many ways, it is a form of guided meditation.

My initial Reiki attunement was a weekend workshop. Day one was pretty much what I expected. We learned the history, guidelines, and principles of the modality. On day two, we reviewed what we'd learned the day before and then we received our attunements.

As we neared the end of the attunement process, it was like my closed eyes were flooded with violet colors like a cloud of that of a lava lamp. It was beautiful and magical, and I'll never forget it. Those colorful clouds have grown and emerged into different colors and combinations of colors over time. I now see images, faces, and things I cannot describe from time to time just by closing my eyes.

I remember being in such disbelief when I got home that night that I asked my husband. "What do you see when you close your eyes?" as if I might have missed this little aspect my entire life. His response was "Darkness," with a very strange look on his face. Well, there you go. I'm not crazy. Well, he might have thought so at the time, but now he comes home from time to time and asks for Reiki. Who knew?

After our attunement ceremony, we participated in a Reiki share. For the first time, this is a mind-blowing experience. At the onset of the process, my hands started to heat up. My intuition had received a total jump start, and I was on high alert. I could feel where our instructor needed attention, and I was guided to return to her shoulder. She later asked who was at my shoulder that had been giving me trouble lately. Amazing!

Then I received Reiki from the others in the class and was amazed at how grounded and relaxed I felt when I was done. Our homework upon leaving class was to perform self-care Reiki daily to fine-tune our craft and prepare to move forward if we wished.

Little did I know that this was just the beginning of the healing process for me, never mind anyone else. I still do my Reiki self-healing most mornings before I get out of bed, and it has served me well. The healing process has been subtle in the short term, but looking back over time, it has been enormous. I can feel physical changes in my digestion when my hands go to my solar plexus and my sacral chakras. My emotions and spiritual growth have increased tenfold since that beautiful day.

Several months later, I received my Reiki II and my sacred symbols. This was another big jump in this sacred realm, which propelled me forward in all other arenas as well. In 2020, I received my Reiki III attunement, otherwise referred to as Reiki master.

I had no intention of going further than Reiki II, to be honest. I was content with where I was, but apparently, the universe had other plans. My Reiki master called me one day and asked if I'd be joining them the next day for the Reiki master attunement. I didn't even know it was happening.

Since the country had shut down and I was not working, I replied that I really couldn't afford it. She continued, "Maybe you can manifest it …"

I replied, "OK, if I come up with the money by morning, I'll be there," silently laughing it off. I jokingly told my husband about the conversation that evening, and we laughed and moved on to the next subject.

The next morning, he asked if I was going to attend. I replied, "Did I manifest 400 dollars in my sleep last night?"

He simply replied, "Just use my card." And here we are. That to me is the universe in action at its best, not only guiding me in the direction of what I want (unknowingly) and need but nudging me to that open door. John's reasoning was "Candy, you started it. You might as well finish it."

That winter, I received my Reiki master teacher training, and that is when I discovered my dream for Reiki. Reiki teaches us how to manage emotions and energy at all levels. It's not about suppressing emotions but coming to terms with our anger, peeling back all the layers to see what the source of the issue is, feeling it fully, and being able to truly let it go for good.

The Reiki principles are a great starting point to help understand what it is all about. These principles are recited daily as part of our self-healing sessions. The original principles are

> Just for today, I will not worry.
> Just for today, I will not be angry.
> Just for today, I will be humble.
> Just for today, I will be honest.
> Just for today, I will be compassionate toward myself and others.

During an attunement, we are encouraged to create our own principles that fit more precisely with our individuality. Mine are

> Just for today, I will not worry, I will not anger.
> Just for today, I will work mindfully and completely.
> Just for today, I will nourish my mind and body.
> Just for today, I will share my gifts with the world, beginning with myself.
> Just for today, I will be kind to all that I meet, especially me.

The Reiki principles, whether the originals or your own, are an amazing way to start your day out on the right foot. I love setting the tone for my day first thing in the morning. I always start with my self-healing practice, and my Reiki principles are how I close out that practice.

My love for Reiki is even with my love for meditation. Being able to combine the two in order to maximize the effects of both makes me even happier. I love to share and spread this calming energy wherever I can. One assists the other and vice versa.

I use my Reiki in so many ways during the day and throughout life. When we moved into our new home, I used it to clear any old energies. When we painted the walls, I painted empowerment symbols on them before painting over them. I use my symbols to bless my food as well as my office and the building I work in every morning. I ask for divine guidance while channeling and creating new meditations and healing activations. I draw an empowerment symbol on my steering wheel before I drive anywhere. I send healing energy to friends, family, acquaintances, and even people I don't know. The possibilities are endless.

Note though that Reiki is a modality of free will, meaning it is considered improper to provide Reiki without permission. A person must be receptive to the energy and the concept. So as practitioners, we must respect others' wishes before sending Reiki whether in person or by distance. If you have no way to obtain this permission, there are a couple of ways to proceed cautiously. First, ask your higher self if the person is receptive. If you see them turn back to you in your third eye, then they are receptive. If they do not acknowledge and move away, then they are not, and it is not advised. Another way is to premise the Reiki energy with the statement "If this energy is not welcomed, may it be recycled back to the earth." I love using this in any distance healing as the earth always needs our help in healing.

It was very soon after I received my Reiki master teacher training that I was approached by an acquaintance to provide her master attunement. I was a little nervous about it as I had not actually done any other attunements myself yet. I felt like I was not practiced enough or worthy of a master's degree at that time.

Once again though, the universe did its work. At the time, she didn't have the money to do so anyway, so we put it off for another time. Then I was guided to call her and offer the attunement at half price two weeks later. I questioned it as I was still a little insecure about it. The answer was an astounding "You need to do this." I called her, and we did it the following weekend.

The whole experience removed any insecurities and reservations I had immediately. Throughout the duration of the morning, we discussed our experiences, beliefs, and love of the craft. In the beginning, she described the strange dream she had had the evening before about some tall, robed people standing around in a circle around a fire. She didn't understand why. Once we finished the physical attunement process, she explained to me that she now understood the dream. As I was sending the sacred symbols to her crown chakra, she saw each of these beings fly into her third eye.

This was the true confirmation that I was not overstepping my authority by doing this Reiki master attunement. Divine reassurance, I love it. This attunement was also when I realized that we all receive and use/perform our Reiki gifts differently.

When being attuned, there is a specific way and order to go about giving a healing session. This is not meant to restrict the practitioner. It is just a good starting point. Intuition and guides will take care of the rest. At that time, I had only performed sessions and attunements exactly as I had learned, and I was intrigued when she informed me that she did the majority of her sessions remotely as in-person sessions for her were very difficult because she would receive a loud buzzing sound that was very distracting. When she did them remotely, she found the buzzing noise was much softer and did not distract her at all.

Soon after, that was when I started receiving messages while performing a Reiki healing session. These messages made no sense to me at all, but once I started to ask my clients, they would know exactly what it meant. That being said, I then decided to ask at the beginning of the session: If any messages came through, would they like to hear them? Some people do and others do not—again, free will here. Always respect the wishes of your client.

I always suggest prior to and after performing Reiki healing, readings, or attunements, be sure to take great care of yourself physically and spiritually. Always be conscious of how much is enough and how much is too much.

I experienced negative physical effects after an intense session when I first started receiving additional information. I always suggest protecting your energy prior to the session either by a white light ritual or other form of ritual protection that resonates with you. I've gotten so I wear bracelets of crystals, which I visualize blocking energy from climbing back up my arms. Always be sure to nourish yourself with good food and rest before and after sessions as well. I've also experienced my back going out several times before I realized what was happening.

If you are attuning multiple people at once, always be very present with your intuition as to what may be too much. Your guides will let you know if you ask. I know we are all here to help others, but as always, we can't help others if we don't help ourselves. If you try to attune too many people in one session, you will drain yourself and not give them the best energy they can receive in their attunement experience. So be aware and be sure to listen to your guides.

Another great thing is that you always have your Reiki abilities with you. So when you are feeling under the weather or just a little run-down, be sure to fall back on your self-healing practice. I do this every morning before I get out of bed and more on days when I'm feeling stressed or unwell in any way. At that moment, you can use your sacred symbols to give yourself energy, strength, or whatever you need at that time.

Just last night, I used it for a headache, and I was able to make it go away without any medications at all, which always makes me happy. I hate taking medications, over-the-counter or otherwise.

There are so many ways we can use Reiki in our lives. We can use it in the traditional manner by balancing the chakras or, as I just mentioned, to help with a headache, stomachache, or something of that sort. We can use it for stress or to calm the energy in a room.

I often use my symbols on the door of my office or the chair a client will sit in. I'll use the empowerment symbol on my steering wheel, my food, my drinks, or my computer screen. I'll bless my technology when recording a meditation or channeled healing. And I'll imagine an emotional symbol over a frantic client's body. I regularly infuse my meditations with Reiki healing energy and state at the beginning of them to just say yes to receive the benefits of the energy, once again allowing choice and free will.

Sending distant energy, prayers, and healing is another way that can really help our world and is so much more effective than people may think. The possibilities are endless, and you will never guess where your next recipient may come from or when. Just the other night, my mom reached out. She explained that she had been fighting a headache for days, and my aunt (who is also a Reiki master) suggested she hold her hands up in front of her eyes.

My mom wrote to me to tell me that it was helping. Of course, I wasn't surprised but also explained she would have even more success if she got her attunement. So we've planned to get her, my brother, and his daughter together some weekend and do all of their attunements. My brother and niece have been talking about it for a while. This is very exciting to me. I can't wait.

There will always be doubters and nonbelievers out there. In fact, a friend is one of them even though he says he isn't. He's told me more than once that he's open-minded, but he never gets anything from it. He'll explain that he's received it from an aunt many times and never feels anything.

Yet I've given him sessions after a back surgery when he's been severely constipated, and I feel and hear things start to get moving as we move down his body. Then he started passing gas and even acknowledged it while it was happening. But since then, he still claims it never works. I don't take this personally. We help in whatever way we can and meet people where they are. Plus, whether he knows it or not, I know it's helping him.

I truly look forward to the day when I can attune my mom, brother, and niece and see what a change it will bring into each of their lives in its unique way for each of them. I know I found healing that I did not know I needed, but I am truly grateful for the opportunity to receive and to give back from that day forward.

What is amazing to me is that even if someone receives their attunement for no other reason than for self-healing, they are still healing the world more than they know because when we heal ourselves, we heal the world. The people around us see that we are different, they feel that we are different, and we shine our light brighter than ever before. This energy is contagious and cannot be resisted by many. When we feel better, those around us do as well.

Reiki can be used in so many ways, and it is different for every person who practices it, whether just for themselves or for others. For me, I start my day with self-healing before I even get out of bed and end my day the same way before I go to sleep. I infuse my food and beverages with Reiki energy. I clear chairs and rooms with Reiki. I empower and protect my car, my home, my family, and all I come in contact with each day by incorporating it into my meditations and my prayers. I've infused these words with Reiki, and I firmly believe that these words come from that higher power and are divinely guided to share with the world.

That in itself is one of my biggest dreams, to share Reiki with the world and bring it to the mainstream, bring it out of the shadows of woo-woo land and into our daily lives. I believe our world has evolved now to a point where the general population is ready, and not only are they ready for it, but they are also in need of it. We need the ability to self-heal from within. We need the ability to join forces and allow our healing energy to create healing change in the world.

This cannot happen with just a few of us. To some extent, that's the beauty of it. We all need to come together and share our power to heal the world. We can heal ourselves and heal the world as a growing and emerging community.

Even though Reiki is a modality of free will, the more of us who share it, the more of us will join. Our love is contagious and can spread just as easily as this virus that has taken over our world. The more we share, the more it catches on.

I believe our world is truly ready for change, but change is not like what we hear about every day from businesses and politicians. I'm talking about a huge change of heart, a change in how we feel about each other. Not just our biological brothers and sisters and friends, I'm talking about our brothers, sisters, friends, and family of a different kind—those whom we have not met yet. I believe the world is ready to love unconditionally. We just don't know how.

I never dreamed of a day when my dad would ask for Reiki healing, never mind receiving an attunement. I never dreamed my husband would be open to the messages I receive from my higher power, but the more we share what we are passionate about, the more others will listen and investigate and join us on this journey to a more conscious world, a world where we all care for each other and live in peace and harmony.

In 1976, a study took place that proved a phenomenon that when 1 percent of a community practiced transcendental meditation (TM), the crime rate was reduced by 16 percent on average. This was named the Maharishi effect. The theory was initially proposed in 1960 by Yogi Maharishi Mahesh, its namesake.

This phenomenon is not limited to just TM. It can be and is used in many forms around the world every day. I belong to an empath group and have several friends who all participate in group prayers and group meditations. We all share a prayer list each week, and all meditate on, pray on, or send healing energy to those on the lists. Some of these groups meet physically, online, or all just join in practice at a certain time of day. There are no set rules. Some will send prayers, others telepathic energy, and others like me, Reiki energy.

It all comes down to the same thing. Sharing love for those around us and those in need—that is what it is all about. There is nothing to be afraid of in these groups. When we are living on purpose for a higher good, then we are always protected and honored for our practice.

6

FEAR AND CREATIVITY

> One of the greatest discoveries a man makes, one of his great surprises, is to find he can do what he was afraid he couldn't do.
> —Henry Ford

When I was growing up, creativity was my thing. I loved to paint and draw, do pottery, build things, and more. I couldn't get enough. In high school, we were required to take one art class in our four-year career. I enrolled in six. I had planned on going to art school when I graduated.

That didn't happen. Back in the day, I would blame that on my boyfriend at that time, who eventually became my husband, father of my two beautiful children, and eventually ex-husband. The reality of the situation is that I was scared.

He didn't want me to go away for four years, so I decided instead I'd go to hairdressing school. Even that didn't happen. Yes, again the fear within me was controlling me. I stayed in our little north-country town and became a store clerk, then a receptionist, and so on.

He and I moved in together and out and in again. We had our issues, to be sure. Eventually, we were married. Two years later, we had our first beautiful girl, and four years after that, we had our second beauty.

During this time though, my creativity had dwindled down to nothing. For some reason, I had let my fears control my entire life. I feared looking different from others. I feared my husband criticizing me. I feared the cost of having any hobbies and the anger I would receive for spending the extra money.

Our marriage ended just before our ten-year anniversary, but I didn't see all of this happen before my eyes. I had not seen how I'd let all that I loved so much go because of my own fears. I look back now and laugh.

Soon after he moved out, I painted the living room with bright pink and black zebra stripes. I'd opened the door that had been hiding all my passions. I will always remember when my current husband and I first got together, he said to me, "I can't wait to see what you blossom into". Sometimes I laugh wondering if this is what he thought that would be.

Even as a health coach, I had times when I thought I wasn't being creative but then realized I really was; it was just in a different way from how I used to be creative. Then I moved to creating events, classes, and workshops. I was doing my own marketing and creating the visual materials for all of that.

I wrote a cookbook and spent a whole year creating new recipes, testing them, and editing them until they were perfect. I did all the photography for that book and had a blast doing it.

I've found that creativity makes my life so much richer, and what that looks like continues to change and evolve every day. Today I am writing this book, which never entered my mind back in those high school days. I play with henna and create new designs. I create jewelry out of crystals. I create new meditations every day, a new altar every week or so, and continue to create new recipes every day.

As I sit here this morning, editing the pages before you, I'm receiving text messages from my second beautiful daughter. This girl has stepped out and done what her mama couldn't do. She went to art school and faced her fears and her anxiety when she moved from a small New Hampshire town to New York City to go to the Fashion Institute of Technology (FIT).

That girl has now graduated with her degree in textiles and started her new job yesterday. She stepped into the world she had been working so hard for. Yet this morning, she is filled with anxiety and fear.

Through her fear in our conversation, I realized we face these fears repeatedly in life. But if we don't get creative and step into our power and our dreams, we will be held back. This morning she is feeling how hard change is. Hopefully, sooner than later, she will feel that it was all worth it. I am so very proud of this girl.

So it makes me wonder. How are you creative in your life? Creativity is actually a big part of our lives, and as a health coach, I consider it as food. Yes, actually a primary food. Primary foods are all the things in life that give us energy or take it away but that we don't put it in our mouths. These primary foods are things like spirituality, relationships, finances, career, home cooking, and creativity, just to name a few. You know, the things in life that light us up or suck us dry.

We all have friends who may not take good care of themselves, but they live life on the edge. They are going all the time, doing amazing things, and living life. You wonder how the heck they do it, living on burgers and fries and hardly any sleep. They are living on primary foods.

I have this friend whom I haven't seen in a while, but she eats terribly. She is picky as heck and eats popcorn for lunch. If you take her out, she asks for a dry burger with no bun and some fries. Yet she and her husband ride their Harleys all over the place, they party all the time, and then they carry crippled people up mountains on the weekends so they can see something they'd never otherwise see.

This is living life on primary foods. Though I don't suggest taking this pattern on in your life by any means, it just goes to show you how primary foods can really enrich our lives, and creativity is a huge one of those primary foods.

I feel our creativity comes from sources. I find the more connected I am to my higher power, the better my creative juices flow. At times, it is so obviously clear that the messages on these pages are channeled information from above, and at those times, I am so honored to bring these messages to you. Other times, when I know that my story can help heal others, that is when I know I am just following my purpose of helping others on this journey we all are trying to figure out.

Take a moment now to think about what creativity you have in your life. How are you creative? That doesn't have to involve a paintbrush or a pencil. It comes in so many forms. It could be as simple as arranging a room or a vase of flowers. It could be creating a nice meal for your family or a loved one. It could be maintaining your yard and making it look perfect. What do you do in your life that you take pride in and enjoy doing?

This is your creativity, and the great thing about creativity is that it's very individual. It's supposed to be. If we all created the same things in the same way, it wouldn't be creative. It would be boring. So take pride in your individual view of the world and create the things that make you happy. Share that with the world because we all need another point of view around us.

That youngest daughter we talked about earlier graduated from the Fashion Institute of Technology this year, and I've so enjoyed watching her journey. It's been amazing to watch her change and evolve throughout her collegiate journey. I can't wait to see exactly where she lands in her creative ventures. There have been and will continue to be highs and lows, but I know she will prevail.

She surprised us during her senior year of high school when she said she wanted to go to art school because throughout high school, everyone would ask her if she was as artistic as her sister. My oldest has some pretty amazing talents as well. She had always resented it a little and gave people an emphatic no. Yet she's the one who took it to another level.

My oldest, on the other hand, is still creative in all her own ways. She is a dental assistant getting ready to go back to school but all about beautiful and healthy teeth. She's a personal trainer and a yoga teacher, and she helps so many people create healthy and beautiful bodies. She empowers and inspires others every single day.

I am so proud of both of my girls and the paths they've chosen, especially all the fears they have faced. When I look at them and back to me, it makes me so proud that they meet the world head-on and create their own dreams. That is what it is all about.

Personally, I feel that creativity is channeled information or downloads. I truly believe that all the inspiration and ideas that we come up with out of the blue really are out of the blue. I profess them to be sent from above.

The key is to act upon all of our creative ideas when we receive them. All too often, we doubt our ideas, our thoughts, and our abilities. We have been told for way too long things like "She's a daydreamer," "Her head in the clouds," and "Come back down to earth." Well, we are now in the age of enlightenment, so these things that used to be thought of as bad things are becoming much more normal and even preferred in our present world.

If we can give ourselves permission, we need to be creative and listen to that creative insight and intuition. We could make so much progress in a more suitable direction in all of our lives.

What do you do when you initially have a great idea for something big? What is your first response? Is it positive or negative? If it is positive, then congratulations. If it is negative, let's turn that around. Can you believe in yourself at this moment, concerning these thoughts and ideas? Can you work toward believing in yourself and believing it to be possible?

Sometimes it takes baby steps. We've been programmed for years that creativity is a bad thing. My daughter Jordan has been dealing with it since she entered college, but she keeps finding her own path. I have no doubt that she will be a success in her field. She has never thought like that. When she decides she wants to do something, she just assumes she will, no questions asked. She may run into those spells of anxiety here and there along the way, but she never gives up on her dreams.

I think we all could take a lesson from the twenty-five-year-old and live a little less in our comfort zone. I assume we don't receive these bright ideas of creative light just so that we can stash them back in the corner of our brains to be forgotten. What would be the point anyway?

Those creative ideas are meant to be birthed and nurtured to maturity. They are meant to come alive and be shared with the rest of the world. We all have different outlooks on all kinds of things in this world. If we all acted on those visionary ideas, can you even imagine how our world could change for the better? Imagine all the options and progress this world would go through.

Lately, I'm trying to be more spontaneous as well and act on my creative juices much quicker than I used to. Just this morning, I thought that I had time to create a meditation before I went to work. Usually, I create them in my mind or on paper throughout the week and then record them on the weekend, but we had a busy weekend and didn't get either done.

So I stepped into my sound room this morning and channeled one into the microphone. Then I even had time to edit and upload it. If I had waited for that more opportune time to do so, I probably would have forgotten the subject I'd thought I should share, and that meditation might have never made its way into the world.

I thoroughly enjoy that whole process, so why do I often put it off? My guess is fear. Fear of rejection maybe. Fear of someone calling me weird? But many have called me weird over the years, and I still keep pushing forward. Who would know what the source of resistance might be? If we want to live our happiest lives, we need to push those lines.

The other thing I love to do is write, just like I'm doing now. Unfortunately, it's often the first thing that gets neglected and pushed out of the way, hence the reason it's taken me years to write this book. But every now and then, I get reminded of the things that are going to get me where I want to be, and if I don't do them, then those goals will never be met.

Just this morning while I was finishing my meditation, I decided to change it up a little and use my manifestation letter space as a free writing activity instead. I remember learning years ago about morning pages by

Julia Cameron. I've always thought it was a great idea but never followed through. This morning, I was inspired to partake. What do you know—all that came up was if you don't write the book, it will never happen. "Write the book, Candy. Just write the book." And here we are. I believe that was a creative way for my higher power to get me back on track. Sometimes just doing something a little out of your ordinary routine can really stir the creative juices a little and keep things interesting.

That one little change in my day got me back on track in telling my story again. It's so important to keep doing what you love, and oftentimes, what you love in one way or another includes some creativity, whether that means it's a creative process like writing or it is a creative process to fit it into your day. Is it a creative process to find a friend to join you in the journey? Creativity comes in so many forms it's almost unimaginable.

Check this out. I just looked down at the clock and noticed it was 2:22. We've talked about my passion for angel numbers already. A quick Google search turned this up: angel number 222 is all about trusting yourself and finding ways to work out your current situation. It emphasizes creativity, and this creativity can lead to further self-discovery. Crazy, right? Those cool little synchronicities are the things that keep me trusting that I'm on the right track and that I should just keep going.

I just finished a five-day manifestation challenge with Master Sri Akarshna, and this morning, he advised smudging the house and office and cleaning up the clutter, things I've done many times. He also said to take a look at your vision board to see if it needs an update. Oh boy, does it! My vision board is in our home office, which I use to work from every day. I hardly ever go there since I took a job outside the home.

What good is a vision board if you never see it? So I stood in front of it for a few minutes and finally decided to bring some of those pictures and images where I could see them all day. I saved them to my lock and home screens on my phone. So every time I pick it up I can see the book I'm writing and the microphone from which I will be speaking to all of you. These are little whims of creativity that have the potential to pay off in some amazingly big ways.

Sometimes even the most creative individuals can have a dry spell, and we may not even realize it. I do find that sometimes when I'm feeling a little blocked with my creative juices, I'll take some time to get back in touch with my higher self. Yes, I literally talk to my higher self and ask. What's my next best step? Word? Task? And so on. I find that if I take some time away and get with friends or colleagues, I can get inspired. A lot of the time, I might be a little overwhelmed by all the tasks before me, and that's what causes me to push off the things I love to do.

I also find that unplugging from the normal daily buzz can do amazing things for my creativity too. Just taking a break from all the notifications on my phone breaks that cycle of always being in demand. I'll go for a walk and take the dog instead of my phone. Go for a hike or get a massage. What would you do?

Being creative shouldn't be a chore. It should be enjoyable and it should flow with ease, so if it's not, then take a break. Forcing the issue will not help. Yet I do find that when you are having trouble in any area of your life, creativity can save the day. Isn't this ironic?

Think about this for a minute. Where in your life are things not going quite as you'd like? Is there an area you are struggling with? Take for example, this morning I met with my health and fitness coach, and prior to our call, I was assessing where I was and had noticed that in the past week, I'd been letting other things get in the way of my workouts.

This is a pattern of mine, and I know that I do well for a few months and then for some reason, I start to let other things take priority over what I really need to accomplish my fitness goals. This was my last call with my coach in my ninety-day program, so how would I keep myself motivated? I am also studying to get certified as a personal trainer, and ironically, I've been letting my study time be one of those things that get in the way. I know—it doesn't make much sense, does it?

So my creative mind decided that this is my opportunity to perfect my personal trainer knowledge and see how I can incorporate it into my own fitness journey. I've decided that this is divine timing for me to step into my own power and create a better connection with this knowledge I'm trying to obtain.

No matter what issue you're dealing with in life, you can use creativity to find a solution. Many times, a nontraditional approach to the situation may be just what is needed.

Raising children, for example. My oldest daughter was, as children go, a pretty easy child. She minded well and followed rules and to this day is so responsible that I often wonder if she has enough fun. I always say she has been a mom since she was four when her sister was born. In fact, she used to make me a little crazy informing me of all the things that her sister needed. I had to remind her often that she did have a mother.

Her sister, on the other hand, was a bit more of a rebel, bucking the system every step of the way. To get where I wanted our end result to be with her, I often had to be creative. The rules had to be a little different from time to time, as was my reaction to some of the things she would come home with, tell me, and so forth. She loved a good shocked reaction, so I learned to dampen that a lot.

I had to think outside my normal range of thinking, or I would lose her in a quick hurry. I remember as a teen she was dating a boy who was already dating someone else. I knew if I told her she couldn't see him, it would be all over. I would lose her. So as much as it broke my heart, I told her I couldn't control who she saw but I believed that she as well as this other girl deserved better than this. He would not be allowed at our house or her at his, but that was all I could do.

She did end that relationship within a month, much to my joy, and she has taken her self-value much more seriously since then as well as that of others. I understand that those are very hard decisions to make, and they are also heartbreaking at the time, but I listened to my intuition and got creative.

Speaking of creativity, she is my girl who followed her creative side into her career. Both of my girls are super creative and artistic, but she's the one who decided to go to school to create. She now has a degree in textiles and is passionate about quality in textiles, the feel of different fabrics, their thread counts, and all that good stuff. She takes her work very seriously and passionately.

Just a twenty-minute conversation with her can teach me so many things I didn't know about materials and fabrics. She loves what she does, and she creates every day in one way or another. She also has been super creative when it comes to her anxiety. When a child moves from a small town in New Hampshire to the Bronx and starts school in Manhattan, she's bound to have a little anxiety. As we discussed earlier, that comes and goes and continues to demand creativity from both of us.

She has made me so proud with the ways she has dug in her heels and pushed herself over the hump some days. This takes true strength, and it makes me smile just thinking about all she's overcome to get what she wants in life.

We all have dilemmas every day, and most of us need a little creativity to maneuver those dilemmas from day to day in order to live our lives how we want to live them, be who we want to be, and shine the way we want to shine.

If you're stuck in a dilemma of your own, take some time for some peace and quiet. Settle into a meditation or just sit quietly in your favorite chair with no distractions. Ask yourself, what is a creative solution to this situation? Then just sit quietly with your eyes closed and see what comes up. If you find your mind won't stop the constant chatter, start to focus on the breath. Just follow it in and out, in and out. This is a simple way to shut that chatter down so that you can hear your own creative mind in action.

Though I encourage sitting in the quiet to do this, if you cannot deal with the silence, then I would suggest using Google to find binaural beats for creativity. These tones will help your mind settle into those creative energies and start the juices flowing.

You can also grab a journal and pen or pencil when you do this. If you have inspiration come up while you're here, you'll want to write it all down as soon as you're done. Be sure to do so because at that time, some of the things that come up may seem insignificant, but you may find out later that it is much more important than you initially thought.

7

ESSENTIAL OILS AND CRYSTALS

> There's an oil for that.
> There's a crystal for that.
> —Unknown

There's no one right tool for everyone on this journey and that is exactly why I have so many to share with you. I am always open to trying something new and following the inspiration that is before me. So as we move forward in this book, we'll touch on several different tools that you may or may not be interested in giving a spin. That's totally OK.

Sometimes when you pick up something new, it just feels good. In others, you get nothing. I have had some tools that did not really feel right when I picked them up for the first time yet a year or two later, they come back into my life with a whole new energy and feeling.

I've had some tools catch me by surprise when they really spoke to me but, at the same time, seemed like nothing I would ever be interested in, and they became something I loved and enjoyed every day of my practice. So as we move through these chapters, take what feels good and go with it and leave what doesn't. You may come back to this at a later date and the other items may have a different feeling. This just means it was waiting for divine timing.

Essential Oils

The use of essential oils originated in ancient India, Persia, and Egypt, to mention just a few. These origins date back to 3000 BCE when botanists and physicians were using them as perfumes and medicines. Hippocrates spent an extensive amount of time studying the effects of these aromatics on the human body.

The Greeks and then the Romans in 70 CE had many aromatic practices and expanded their application and uses of the oils to bathing and dressing their beds with them along with the usual bodily perfumes. The Romans were in love with frankincense to the extent that an entire trade system was built for it. This went on to become the Arabian Peninsula to the Mediterranean ports called the Frankincense Road.

Fast-forward to the twentieth century, when the West became fascinated with the use of essential oils for aromatherapy and more. Businesses were built on the production of these oils for perfumes and medications. Today, well over one hundred types of essential oils are in the marketplace. Yet frankincense remains a favorite of them all.

At this moment, the subject may seem a little misplaced, but once you dip your toes into the world of essential oils, you will realize they have a bit of a seductive capacity to them. There is a deep piece of nature to them and a true link to the spiritual world. They can ground us or lift us up and many other uses in between.

My introduction to essential oils was years ago when I was new to health coaching and new to Crohn's disease. Honestly, I thought it would be a good addition to my health coaching business at the time. I dabbled in them for several years. I found certain oils that helped my digestive health, my pain, and my stress. I found oils that helped me settle into my meditations and different ones for different meditations. I'm thrilled to share that information with you now.

The more I learn about essential oils, the more I fall back on them regularly. No matter what is happening in my life, physically, emotionally, and spiritually, there is an essential oil I can use to help.

Body

Physically, essential oils can heal our bodies from simple things like bug bites and bee stings to burns, cuts, and scars. I do remember a day when I was kind of excited when I got a bee sting to go try my lavender and see if it really did relieve the sting. It did. That might have been a good sign that I was hooked and obsessed.

I use an oil called DigestZen on my belly or in my water when I have an upset stomach, on my throat when I have indigestion or heartburn, or under my cheekbones when I have a sinus headache. It still amazes me from time to time how well it works. It's such a simple and natural solution to so many things.

When using essential oils topically, you always want to be careful. Some oils are considered to be hot oils, meaning they can burn your skin. A solution here is to always dilute them with a carrier oil. A carrier oil can be any good-quality oil that you would cook with like olive oil, avocado oil, or even coconut oil. I use liquid coconut oil, jojoba oil, and others.

You especially want to do this if applied to the elderly or children as their skin is much more sensitive. The carrier oil serves another purpose as well. It helps hold the oil to the skin longer for better absorption. Essential oils in their pure form evaporate quickly and sometimes do so before they can fully be absorbed into the skin.

I've used peppermint for burns, fevers, fatigue, and hot flashes. Past Tense is my go-to for headaches, and I am the queen of headaches from various sources. I've been so grateful to have Roman chamomile for a bout of hives and arborvitae for an ingrown toenail. I love lavender or Holy Basil for sleep and when I'm studying for a test or exam, I use vetiver and lavender for better retention.

I can't even count the number of physical uses for essential oils, but this is nothing compared to the emotional connections that oils will open in your world.

Emotions

When I discovered the deep connection between our bodies and our emotions, I was blown away. I spent a year noticing every time I had a physical injury or pain, doing my research to see what the emotional connection was and did that make sense to me.

The truth is every time I did. The information was always on point. This all took place during the 2020 COVID-19 shut down. At this time, I was in a new home, in a new town, and had no job other than selling essential oils, of course. One day, I had a package delivered. I went out to meet the driver, and when I stepped down off the small stone wall, I rolled my ankle. Not only did I roll my ankle, I rolled my whole entire leg and went down face-first in the driveway. My face hit the dirt, and my glasses went flying.

As the driver came around the back of his truck, I was getting up off the ground, with dirt and blood running down my face. I was so embarrassed. He was shocked and just wanted to help, and I wanted to die. I then hobbled back into the house and put my foot up. A couple hours later, I went to make dinner, and I couldn't stand on that foot. Well, great. So I took myself to urgent care and had a severely sprained ankle.

The whole thing seemed so strange though, like it all had happened in a fog. So I looked it up. The emotional connection to the ankle refers to flexibility related to the future—stubborn or wounded.

I had been home for some time, trying to make my health coaching business successful in this tiny little town of 1,300 people in the middle of a pandemic. I was certainly stubborn and didn't want to give up but, at the same time, was also feeling wounded because I really wanted my business to be a success. I really wanted to help people feel better, and how would I be able to do that behind some desk somewhere? I mean, this was my calling. Wasn't this why I'd lost that job a few years earlier? To go live my purpose.

The oils prescribed for stubbornness were wintergreen or oregano. On the wounded end of things, helichrysum, manuka, jasmine, deep blue, and hope were suggested. I believe I made a roller of all of these that I had and applied it to my ankle several times per day. Within a week, I needed my splint no longer. This was a great thing because I'd taken a new job in retail and needed to be on my feet all day.

A couple of weeks earlier, while swapping over laundry. I swear, a towel reached out and grabbed my pinkie finger and yanked it so hard I thought I'd cry. The results I brought up were hiding, helpless, and purposeless. Yup, that was exactly how I felt. I was resisting going back out into the world, feeling helpless because I had no paycheck and my husband was supporting us both and our whole life. I felt totally purposeless because I'd wanted so badly to coach, teach, and help people, but now I had to go get another job that I had no passion for.

The oils prescribed here were cassia, black pepper and lavender, clove, ginger, Roman chamomile, and frankincense. I made a roller of a variety of these oils and before I knew it I was feeling better about my situation and the opportunities that I knew were out there. Can you see where I'm headed now? Can you see the connection already between the physical, the emotional, and the spiritual?

Spiritual

I've used essential oils for my meditations for years and have found they can be very helpful not only to settle into that peaceful place I'm looking for when in meditation, but also to bring me to a different level of spiritual connection.

I've used wood oils like arborvitae for grounding and angelica for a more heightened Akashic experience. I've used blends of woods and flowers to feel a beautiful sense of calm. I found a great book, *Gifts of the Essential*

Oils by Adam Barralet and Vanessa Jean Boscarello Ovens,[6] which made me realize what an array of roles these oils can play in our spiritual journeys and our conscious ascension. Adam also has a YouTube channel, and I love all his videos.

Throughout this book, they discuss the origins of each oil, its best properties, its gifts, affirmations, and combinations with certain purposes. I've thoroughly enjoyed this book and still have barely dipped my toes in the water. What I have indulged in has been very rewarding indeed. It's also a truly beautiful book to indulge in visually as well.

Among their formulations, there are specific blends for the healing and balancing of each of the main chakras. For the root chakra, they recommend blending vetiver, black pepper, cedarwood, and cinnamon bark. For the sacral chakra, jasmine, tangerine, sandalwood, and vanilla. The solar plexus chakra likes ginger, fennel, lemongrass, melissa, and wintergreen. As for the heart chakra, ylang-ylang, geranium, lime, marjoram, and thyme are suggested. For the throat chakra, call in Roman chamomile, cypress, eucalyptus, and rosemary. The third eye is activated by juniper berry, basil, peppermint, spearmint, and star anise. The crown chakra opens to the powers of lavender, frankincense, and Siberian fir. As you can see the combinations and options are endless.

I've enjoyed their assistance with Akashic records and calling in archangels, and my new moon and full moon rituals have been richer and deeper with the assistance of my oils. The great thing is there really are no rules with these beautiful oils. I love diving into the suggested formulas and potions and playing with them. I also love to use them intuitively.

There's something to be said about trusting my gut first thing in the morning to decide which oil or oils will serve me best throughout my day. You can start the same way, with just one oil to start with. Pick one up that just feels good to you. You can diffuse them, wear them, and even add them to foods if you have quality, pure, and safe essential oils.

As mentioned, I started out thinking they may be a good addition to my business, but eventually, I found a passion to learn and experience them in as many ways as I could. Then in 2020 when the country shut down and I was restricted to my home, it was there for me, and they became my job and my passion for the next few years.

That gave me the time and focus to dig in deep and discover everything I could about all of them I could get my hands on. It was amazing to me how much fun I had with them, trying to make a living selling them online, doing cooking classes with them, and using them in any way I could. I had no idea at the time how much healing I would receive with these simple little oils.

It's also amazing the number of different options that become available when you delve into the world of essential oils. You don't have to just rely on the sacred oils that have come down through history like frankincense, myrrh, hyssop, and rose. There are a multitude of oils out there and even more combinations that can be used for different goals and outcomes.

If you want to delve deeper into the world of essential oils, I recommend doing some research. There are some really great quality oils out there and some that have been adulterated and watered down. I also suggest researching the sourcing of your oils. There is a dark side to the essential oil business, and that includes some not-so-humane business practices. Be sure to buy a brand that reinvests in their farmers and takes care of their people. Choose a company with a good moral compass.

I, to this day, still love to dig in and play with my oils for a multitude of different things, from a physical ailment and a much-needed mindset adjustment to a super-deep meditation practice. I never stop learning about all they can do for me, and as long as you go with a quality and reliable brand, I believe you will too.

For the Love of Crystals

My crystals are another tool with which I connect every day. When I first discovered them, I instantly fell in love. I remember the first time I walked into this cute little metaphysical shop and from the doorway I could see a piece of sparkling lepidolite in the next room. I knew at that moment I would be going home with it that day. I also found a lava-rock turtle that day, which I instantly knew was meant for my oldest daughter. She has always loved sea turtles, and it was calling her name. I had it at my home for months before I decided to bring it to her. The day I did, I couldn't decide when I would bring it over until I was sitting at the traffic light and just knew at that moment that now was the time. When I got to her apartment, she wasn't home. I was disappointed but left it on her doorstep and went off to see my girlfriends. Sitting at my friend's house, I got a call from her. I picked up the phone, and she was crying. "Mom, is this turtle from you?"

"Yes," I said. She replied, "Oh my god, it's beautiful. I have had the worst day, and this just made it all better." There's just something about crystals that I truly connect with, and I know I'm supposed to share them with the world.

That piece of lepidolite I had to have that day? Well, I brought it home and looked it up, and it turns out it's the perfect crystal for a Libra. That's me. It's used for harmonizing body, mind, and soul. It's great for relieving stress and anxiety and is an ally in times of change. It soothes the nervous system, strengthens immunity, and allows you to face growth with power and confidence. It also helps connect you to your higher self. It's truly one of my favorites.

I always have crystals on my altar, but on most days, I carry them myself or wear them on jewelry. Some mornings, depending on how I'm feeling, I will hold a certain crystal to assist with my energy for the day.

Sometimes that means dispelling some negative energy with some selenite if my normal palo santo smudge doesn't feel appropriate. On most days, I stand before my crystals and intuitively decide what I will carry with me for that day. Some days I will be inspired to take more than one piece of a crystal because someone else will need some that day. This is why I often purchase multiples of the same crystal because more times than not, I'm guided that someone else will need it just as much as me on that day.

I never know who, but I always know it will happen. Inevitably, by the end of the day, I've discovered just who that stone was meant for. I've had many clients whose day was changed by a tiny little piece. Isn't it amazing how a little gesture can make such a difference in the world?

I remember one client in particular came into my office for her first visit. I already had three crystals set out for her to choose from. After she spent some time telling me why, she broke into tears. This was supposed to be her time. But in the past week, her daughter had gotten a divorce and moved back into the house with her teenage children and her two dogs.

This woman and I had an instant connection. She reminded me of my mom in stature, in wellness (or lack of), and in her demeanor. At the end of her visit, I asked her to choose the stone that she resonated with. She chose a small piece of agate. I then told her that agate is a calming and grounding stone that can help bring some balance into your life and may even encourage communication of truths.

She looked at me and said that it gave her the chill. This lovely lady excelled at our program, and throughout the process, she became even closer with her daughter. On our last visit, she told me that she carries that stone with her everywhere she goes. That made my heart melt.

The first historical knowledge of crystals comes from the ancient Sumerians (c. 4500 to 2000 BC), one of the earliest civilizations, who used crystals in their healing rituals and for inlays in their finest artwork. Lapis lazuli and serpentine were just two of their favorites.

Lapis lazuli is actually one of my favorites and is another that I've been guided to over time. One evening, a friend and I were having dinner and chatting away about crystals, and she stopped mid-sentence and said, "I'm getting lapis lazuli for you." I'd never heard of it at the time. So I went home and ordered some and have since acquired some more. I just love it and I love how it makes me feel. It increases self-knowledge and awareness of one's own thoughts and can help you to trust your inner self. It has assisted me on my higher-self journey for quite some time now. Because of its deep-blue color, lapis lazuli works wonders with the throat chakra and the third-eye chakra. Both of these chakras are represented by blue and purple shades and pertain to elements of self-expression and spiritual connection.

The link between humans and lapis lazuli stretches back more than 6,500 years. It's been treasured by the ancient Mesopotamians and Egyptians and throughout China, Greece, and Rome.

Serpentine is an earthing stone and also opens new pathways for kundalini energy. It aids in meditation and enhances spiritual exploration. Serpentine assists in the retrieval of wisdom, helping to regain memory of past lives.

Serpentine is associated with the heart chakra. This green stone can assist with healing problems within the heart and lungs and boost energy, and it is an excellent stone for cellular regeneration. It encourages us to make contact with the elemental beings as the members of the devic realm resonate with this energy.

Crystals can be used for spiritual, emotional, and physical healing. Just as everything around us, every crystal carries a different vibration. This may seem odd to many, but yes, all matter has a vibration, a movement, a flow of sorts. Yes, even stones or crystals. When you look up crystals in the dictionary, you'll find it referred to as a solid whose atoms are arranged in a highly ordered repeating pattern. Scientists say atoms vibrate, rotate, and move from place to place. The molecules in your pencil, your paper, and even your crystals are in motion right now. Matter exists on earth in three forms: solid, liquid, and gas. These three forms are called the three states of matter. Crystals are of solid form. All the molecules in a crystal vibrate at the same rate, creating a powerful synchronization and a really stable frequency.

Holding crystals or placing them on your body is thought to promote physical, emotional, and spiritual healing. They do this by positively interacting with your body's own energy field or chakra. While some crystals are said to alleviate stress, others can improve concentration or creativity. Still others can help ground us, elevate our mood, help us concentrate, or motivate us.

My brother one evening was simply meditating on his rose quartz skull as he held it in his hands in front of him. As he became more focused and connected, he suddenly felt a jolt of pain shoot down his arm from his shoulder. This startled him, and he quickly set the stone down. He didn't know what to think and was rather shocked.

He had been having pain in his shoulder for months and had finally decided to go see the doctor about it. The surprise was though that, after this event, he had no more pain in his shoulder. The rose quartz had pulled the pain from his shoulder, and it has never returned. He canceled his appointment with the doctor soon after. Each crystal has a slightly different geometric pattern, and many of these patterns can also be found within our cells, organs, and bodily systems. This is likely why they can be of such great assistance to us.

I do intend to borrow his skull someday soon as I'm very curious. I myself have a lot of shoulder pain, as does my sister. I believe there is some past-life connection to this pain as my father has it and all of us three children have it in our right shoulder. Wouldn't it be great if our crystals could be the solution for all of us? To me, this physical manifestation is something of emotional origin back in our lineage somewhere.

Cleansing and charging your crystals

I once had a quartz pendant that I just loved. It always gave me such calmness and connected to my spirituality. It just made me feel good. One day I removed it before getting in the shower and set it down on the sink. The second it hit the sink, it broke in half, and it didn't even hit the surface hard at all. I couldn't believe it. It had hit so lightly but broke right in half.

Crystals can break when they become overcharged with energy or if they become full. This can happen if you work very frequently with a crystal or if it has been exposed to too much sunlight for an extended period of time. When a crystal becomes overcharged or full, its structure becomes unstable, and it may fracture or shatter. Therefore, it is important to clear your crystals. There are several ways to care for your crystals so they can continue to help you long-term.

I love to clear and charge my crystals by the full moon. On a full moon, I will gather my crystals and put them outside to be cleared and charged. Part of charging your crystal is clearing its energetic slate—hence why we refer to charging crystals as clearing them. It's all the same thing. We want to remove any residual energy from prior use so as to start clean and clear and not overload them. I like the full moon for this because that is also how I work with the full-moon energy for my own clearing and charging rituals.

Other ways to charge your crystals may include soaking them in moon water (water charged by the full moon). Some crystals are softer and won't do well in the water, so be careful with this one. Selenite is one that may dissolve over time with water exposure. You can bury them in the ground or in salt, or you can cleanse them with a breath of intention. Just hold your crystals in your hand, intend to clear them with your breath, and then breathe over them. This is great for healers who use crystals regularly and need more frequent care. I also will clear crystals with some Reiki energy when working with a crystal healing grid. I simply state, "I clear this grid of everything but love and use my sacred symbols on them." You can also contact your spirit guides and ask for their assistance. That is the beauty of working with crystals: you can choose what feels right to you at any time and place.

I look at charging my crystals as thanking them for all of their assistance by releasing them from the energies of the past. They will thank you for it with continued service for the higher good. My crystals bring me so much happiness in so many ways. They raise my vibration, change my mood, help me settle into meditation, and discover solutions to my problems. They also just bring me true joy from their pure natural beauty. I have crystals in all the rooms in my home, in and around my plants, and beside my bed. I carry them with me daily and give them to others when they are in need.

8

NUMEROLOGY AND ANGEL NUMBERS

A number sequence that contains a repeated series and spiritual significance

From the time I first entered the metaphysical world, I'd heard about the significance of numbers and how and where they turn up in our lives. I remember thinking, hmmm, I just don't see it. I never noticed anything of interest, significance, or even coincidence.

Then one day as I was driving my commute north listening to Gabrielle Bernstein's book "The Universe has your back"[7], I'd listened to her experiences with angel numbers and was very intrigued. Just as I got to work, I asked my spirit guides to give me a sign if this was something of significance.

The next thing I knew, I started seeing the number 111 everywhere—on license plates, on receipts, and even in the time of day. It became so frequent that I couldn't ignore it. Intrigued, I began researching angel numbers and numerology, discovering a fascinating world of symbolism and guidance.

Angel numbers such as 111 are said to be messages from the spiritual realm, offering insights and guidance in various aspects of life. Each number carries a unique energy and meaning, and the more I paid attention, the more I noticed patterns and synchronicities.

Numerology, a broader system that assigns significance to numbers based on their vibrational energies, further deepened my understanding. It involves interpreting personal numbers like life path and destiny numbers to gain insights into one's life purpose and challenges.

This journey into numerology and angel numbers has brought a new layer of awareness and guidance to my life. It's a reminder that the universe communicates with us in mysterious ways, and there's often more to the seemingly mundane than meets the eye.

That experience with the repeated ones, especially 11.11 and 1.11, seemed like a powerful and synchronistic moment. The fact that it happened while I was settling into my work adds a layer of significance to it. It's fascinating how these numbers, often referred to as angel numbers, can serve as signs or messages from the universe.

The interpretation of 11.11 indicating guidance from a higher power and a connection to the universe aligns with your experience of embarking on a new journey of self-discovery. It's incredible how these subtle signs can offer insight and reassurance during pivotal moments in our lives.

The recurrence of numbers in sequence on most days further underscores the idea that there might be a greater cosmic communication happening. It's a beautiful reminder that the universe is always in dialogue with us, guiding us on our paths. Have you noticed any specific themes or patterns associated with numbers in your life?

Even though some may attribute it to a trained awareness, the sheer magnitude and variety of occurrences I've described, especially beyond the clock, tell me a more profound connection truly exists. It's moments like that which make the mystical aspects of life truly captivating.

Each number indeed carries its unique symbolism even in its singular form.

- Ones are new beginnings and creation.
- Twos symbolize duality.
- Threes embody creativity.
- Fours represent hard work.
- Fives indicate change and challenges.
- Sixes focus on relationships.
- Sevens symbolize contemplation and restraint.
- Eights signify prosperity and abundance.
- Nines embody completion and compassion.
- Zeroes represent cycles and infinity.

The origins of numerology date back to 500 BC, and its popularization by Pythagoras showcases its longstanding presence and influence. It's fascinating how these ancient practices continue to resonate with people today, offering guidance and insight into the complexities of life.

Discovering your life path number and destiny number can indeed be a captivating journey. Have these numbers influenced your perspective or decisions in your life?

Numerology operates on the premise that everything emits energetic frequencies, including numbers, letters, colors, and shapes. Each of these elements carries a unique meaning and vibration. Numerologists believe that birthdates and names, in particular, hold significant energetic importance for each individual.

By assigning numerical values to letters and analyzing birthdates, numerology seeks to unveil insights into an individual's personality, life path, and potential challenges or opportunities. It is a practice that explores the energetic resonance of elements in our lives.

As we delve into numerology, the concept of angel numbers naturally emerges. Rooted in numerology, angel numbers introduce a spiritual and divine dimension. They are viewed as messages from the spiritual realm, offering guidance and insight into one's life journey.

A life path number serves as the initial step in the practice of numerology, often referred to as a master number, expression number, or destiny number. It's a soul-chosen number that plays a pivotal role in facilitating spiritual growth. While various methods exist for calculating this number, this book will utilize the simplified approach based on one's birthdate.

For instance, taking the birthday 10/08/1970, you would add up all the digits and then reduce the total to a single digit. In this example, 1+0+0+8+1+9+7+0=26 further reduces to 2+6=8. This resultant single-digit number becomes a guiding force, offering insight into oneself and potential paths. It becomes a valuable tool for decision-making in various aspects of life.

Numerology encompasses different forms, all stemming from the foundational principle that numbers and letters possess unique energetic connections to each other and to the divine. The life path number, derived from such calculations, unveils a personalized guide for self-discovery and understanding.

Vedic numerology, the oldest system from which many others have derived, maintains a profound connection with astrology, emphasizing the influence of planets on our world. In the Vedic practice, individuals are assigned three distinct numbers: psychic number, destiny number, and name number.

The psychic number reflects how we perceive ourselves and the world. Ranging from one to nine, it is calculated by reducing the day of birth to a single digit. Using the previous example of 10/08/1970, the calculation results in a psychic number of 8. This number becomes a key element in Vedic numerology, offering insights into one's self-perception and worldview.

The destiny number in Vedic numerology provides insights into how we are perceived by the world and our fate. Similar to the calculation of the psychic number, the destiny number is derived by adding up all the digits of the entire birthdate and reducing it to a single digit. In the example given, the destiny number is also 8.

Moving on to the name number, it signifies our destiny or life purpose. This calculation involves assigning a numerical value between one and eight to each letter of the full name as stated on the birth certificate. The values of all the letters are then summed up and reduced to a single digit, unveiling a unique and personalized number that reflects the life purpose or destiny associated with the name.

When calculating your destiny number, these numbers correlate with the following letters:

1	A	I	J	Q	Y
2	B	C	K	R	
3	G	L	S		
4	D	M	T		
5	N	E			
6	U	V	W	X	
7	O	Z			
8	F	H	P		

In my case, Candace Marie Holmes, Candace becomes 2 + 1 + 5 + 4 + 1 + 2 = 20, Marie becomes 4 + 1 + 2 + 1 + 5 = 13, Holmes becomes 8 + 7 + 3 + 4 + 5 + 3 = 30. Then we add those totals, 20 + 13 + 30 = 63, which then reduces to a single digit: 6 + 3 = 9. Everyone's numbers are different, so go ahead and do your numbers and then you can reflect below as to their meaning.

1. Leader: Confident, ambitious, and independent. Challenges include the need to learn how to lose gracefully.
2. Peacemaker: A mediator seeking balance and harmony. Challenges may involve hesitancy, insecurity, and indecisiveness.

3. Creator: expressive and creative, charming, and entertaining. Challenges include potential pessimism, boredom, vanity, and jealousy.
4. Steady: Stable, solid, grounded, and reliable. Challenges involve vulnerability to life's challenges, inflexibility, and stubbornness.
5. Free: Individualistic, adaptable, and spontaneous. Challenges include potential unreliability, flightiness, irresponsibility, and selfishness.
6. Homemaker: Family-oriented, responsible, nurturing, and compassionate. Challenges may include tendencies toward neediness, temperamental behavior, codependency, and neglect of self-care.
7. Philosopher: Practical and esoteric, combining logic with intuition. Challenges include potential argumentativeness and judgmental tendencies.
8. Balance: Successful, focused, with a strong work ethic. Challenges involve potential materialism, impatience, pushiness, and control issues.
9. Humanitarian: Generous, unselfish, and loving. Challenges may include aimlessness, low self-esteem, and feelings of unfulfillment.

This breakdown provides a valuable resource for individuals to explore and reflect on the qualities associated with their life path numbers. It allows for a deeper understanding of strengths and potential areas for personal growth.

The perspective that angels are perceived as more approachable intermediaries between humans and the divine, making communication more relatable, is an interesting and comforting concept. Angel numbers, in this context, become a symbolic language thought which divine guidance is conveyed in a manner that resonates with individual experiences.

Acknowledging the personal and situational variations in the meanings of angel numbers is a crucial point. The fluidity of interpretation allows for a more dynamic and personalized connection between individuals and the messages they receive through these numbers. It emphasizes the idea that the divine communicates with each person in a way that is uniquely tailored to their circumstances and needs. I certainly have found this to be true for me.

The other day, my brother reached out to let me know that he'd received a promotion. He has been going above and beyond the call of duty for years, and I had encouraged him to push back because I felt that his company was taking advantage of his generosity and good work ethic. The moment I received his text message, I looked at the clock and it was 11:11. The recurring appearance of 11:11 in your life, especially during significant moments like my brother's job announcement, is a powerful and personal experience. Many people explore the energetic significance of 11:11 and how energy tends to evolve as sequences build. Let's explore that some more.

- 11:11 is often seen as a gateway or opening to higher spiritual awareness. It's a reminder that your thoughts and intentions are aligning with your spiritual path. The repeating 1s amplify the energy, emphasizing the power of manifestation and the alignment of mind, body, and spirit.
- 22:22 this sequence carries the energy of balance and harmony. It suggests that your dreams and aspirations are aligning with divine timing. The repeating 2s emphasize partnerships, cooperation, and the importance of maintaining balance in different aspects of life.
- 33:33 represents the energy of the ascended masters and signifies divine protection and guidance. It's associated with compassion, healing, and the manifestation of positive outcomes. The repeating 3s intensify the influence of spiritual growth and assistance from higher realms.
- 44:44 this sequence brings the energy of stability, support, and manifestation of your goals. It's a sign that your angels and guides are actively assisting you in bringing your dreams into reality. The repeating 4s enhance the energy of foundation and grounded progress.

- 55:55 symbolizes significant and positive changes on the horizon. It's a message that transformation is occurring, and your angels are supporting you through the process. The repeating 5s emphasize freedom, adaptability, and the ability to embrace change with confidence.
- 66:66 encourages shifts and change toward more balance and alignment from a materialistic perspective to a more spiritual one.
- 77:77 is most often a sign to align with those energies of love, understanding, and empathy to bring positive transformation to your relationships.
- 88:88 is always a reminder of the abundance around you and is on its way. It is often pointing to and preparing you for the amazing opportunities ahead.
- 99:99 signifies and recognizes the changes and the personal development you've been working on.

As you've observed with 11:11, these sequences indeed carry forward and intensify the energetic messages, providing a deeper and more profound connection with the spiritual realm. It's a beautiful way to feel guided and supported during key moments in life. If just these numbers have piqued your interest, I suggest you follow your heart and follow where the numbers lead you.

9

OTHER SPIRITUAL TOOLS

> Breathe in deeply and let your life unfold.
> —April Peerless

Prayer

When I was a child, prayer was something you had to do and something that required a specific way. There were rules and guidelines as to how you should and shouldn't pray. As an adult, I've concluded that prayer looks different to every single one of us and there is no right or wrong way to do this. In those childhood days, I saw prayer as the rules I had to follow to thank God for what I had and ask for what I wanted.

It is defined as an act of communication by humans with the sacred or holy—God, the gods, the transcendent realm, or supernatural powers. Found in all religions at all times, prayer may be a group or personal act utilizing various forms and techniques. This really reflects how I see prayer in my world today.

I think as we are raised in a certain religious order, we may be forced to fall within the thinking of others before ours. I feel like this may limit us at times in our ascension process. In fact, that is really the purpose of this book: to share with the world all the tools available to us in order to find our own ascension and our own higher consciousness.

I consider prayer another amazing tool given to us to communicate and connect with our higher power, our guides and angels, and our higher self. I also think this is the point where we acknowledge that there is something bigger than ourselves and truly accept that as reality. When we pray in any way, we are connecting to that thing that is bigger than ourselves even if we cannot fully explain that form, energy, or vision of what that is. It is what we believe and know within ourselves.

The biggest and greatest thing about prayer is we can do it anywhere, anytime, as long as and in whichever form we wish to do so. We do not need to get down on our knees and fold our hands, though this is certainly an option. We can also intend our thoughts to be a prayer. I silently pray throughout my day. I pray out loud after my meditation every morning. I think a prayer of gratitude at bedtime and when I open my eyes each morning. I send out prayers of peace every morning after my Merkabah meditation (the unity prayer). I create crystal grids and attach a prayer of healing for people and the world. Prayer can truly take thousands of different forms and look different to everyone.

Angels, Guides, and Animal Spirits

Angels and guides are where I direct many of my prayers every day. I start many of my prayers with "Angels and guides of the highest and best power". The highest and best power portion helps weed out any angels or guides not of such. When we request only that, then only that will step in.

There are angels and guides with less-than-honorable intentions, so it is wise to include such discernment. This way, you will only invite higher power and highly intentioned helpers on your journey.

We all have our own personal angels and guides, and we also may share some of both. Some are sent to assist just you and others will assist many. Some people are guided by ancestors, friends, and even pets that have passed on.

During a past life reading a couple of years ago, my friend explained to me that my guides had been off over her right shoulder. She asked me if I knew of a cat named Shorty. I replied yes, I used to have a gray-and-white cat named Shorty. She then informed me that he was one of my guides. I was shocked. Really? A cat?

At that time, I had no idea that was even a possibility. Since then, I have learned that animal spirits are also here to help us in our ascension journey. This is where spirit animals and animal totems come into play.

Once upon a time, when my husband was not so sure about all my spiritual mumbo jumbo (as I imagined him thinking), I would pull an animal spirit oracle card for him each morning. I thought this might be more relatable for him.

I kept doing it even though I didn't know if he was thinking I was crazy or not. One day, he came home and said, "So I've been thinking about your cards," and went on to tell me the reason why. The cards had pointed some things out to him in his life, and he had truly made the connection.

I have also learned to pay attention to the animals that turn up in my life. When we first moved to our home in Southern New Hampshire, I was on a walk one day all by myself. The road across from our house goes through a nice little neighborhood and then extends into a more wooded and remote area for about a mile.

As I was walking on this warm morning, suddenly, a large wolf gracefully ran across the road in front of me about twenty yards away. It was startling yet it was almost surreal. He was there and he was gone out of and back into the swamp on an elegant and majestic gate; he was gone. Once I passed where he crossed my path, I turned around to see where he'd gone, and to be sure, he wasn't behind me. I couldn't shake the feeling that this was so strange and felt so magical and that there was a reason he had crossed my path that morning.

Once I got home, I did some research. The wolf symbolizes an intriguing mix of power, loyalty, guardianship, teamwork, and wildness. At this time in our lives, John and I were pretty much all each other had. We'd moved to this little town in the middle of a pandemic. He had lost both of his parents, and I had moved away from mine. We had no friends here, and no one was willing to invite anyone, given the state of the world. We were truly loyal to each other and have always been our own team. This to me was reminding me of that—reminding me that we were a powerful team and we could accomplish anything together. Many cultures traditionally value the wolf as a powerful guiding force. Wolves are extremely intuitive and have an almost supernatural instinct that can detect dangerous situations. I felt no danger that day as I looked behind me. I was more interested in seeing if I had imagined the whole thing.

As for my own cat as my spirit guide, the gray cat symbolizes "very positive characteristics such as independence, liberty, spiritual enlightenment, intuition, balance, and hope."

Oracle Cards

As I mentioned before when I was pulling cards for my husband, I would use Animal Spirit cards, which are just one form of oracle cards. Oracle cards are one of the very first tools I worked with as I started to delve into my spiritual inquisition.

Oracle cards are a set of divinatory cards that are used for personal exploration and ritual, usually created by someone with some spiritual history or gifts themselves. When I first picked up my first oracle deck, it was what felt comfortable to me as I was just beginning to explore the metaphysical world as I did not know it at the time.

It felt like it was a safe way for me to play and see what this world was all about. I immediately felt a connection with this first deck of Moonology cards, which is a deck of oracle cards in all stages of the moon. I was continually amazed with the accuracy of them every time I used them. I would simply ask the cards each morning, "What do I need to know for my highest and best good today?"

I then graduated to a deck from Collette-Baron Reed and then I fell in love with Rebecca Campbell's "Work Your Light" deck. I used these cards most days for over a year. I know these cards helped me put down the wine bottle and step into my own power.

I will say this didn't happen overnight, but those cards kept at me until I truly listened. I can't tell you how many times I pulled the niggle card the morning after drinking too much wine. This card says, "Trust the Niggle." What is that niggling feeling trying to tell you? It was trying to tell me to put down the bottle, but I was not listening. Even after I did notice, I would pull it repeatedly. "Candy, you're not listening."

The card continues, "That niggling feeling. That annoying, niggling feeling. That inconvenient, annoying, niggling feeling. Try as you might, it's there. And it isn't going anywhere. Most people spend years ignoring their niggling feelings. Throwing their best dollops of stubbornness, ego, and post-rationalization to numb them out. It's exhausting. And until you face the niggle, life just throws you more bait to awaken it. To draw your attention to the light within you that is bursting to come out. The niggle is an arrow pointing to what is standing in your way—the relationship, the conversation, the decision, the shift that needs to be made, the stone in your shoe.

"Often, we feel the niggling feeling in our body first. Many people think that intuition is something from the higher realms, but in fact, it is the body that is the intuitive one, working through our senses to deliver vibrational information. It takes just a moment every day to scan your body to receive intuitive intelligence and act on it quickly.

"You are being called to face the niggle now. If you don't face it, the universe will throw something much bigger and more obvious in your path. And then you will likely regret that you didn't answer the niggle in the first place. I know it's scary, but you are safe. Answer the niggle now." Eventually, I listened, and luckily, I did before something worse happened. To this day, I still love her cards and her books. They are one of my all-time favorites. More recently I've been using the Isis cards by Alana Fairchild. I was guided to these cards over the course of events. I have the pocket edition and, for a while, carried them with me much of the time. I just love how these cards feel in my heart. This is another thing that was recommended to me by my friend and boss, and her guidance has always served me well.

Activating the Merkabah

I've recently taken a break from all my oracle cards and any other form of divination as I've been working with my higher self-connection. As I mentioned earlier, in one of my first healing sessions, my healer saw a Merkabah. At the time, I had no idea what that was. I did look it up at the time but never really pursued it any further than that.

The Merkabah is a piece of sacred geometry. Sacred geometry is the belief that basic properties of the universe can be calculated into simple shapes and patterns. It is believed that this geometry is centered on a grid of overlapping circles referred to as the Flower of Life.

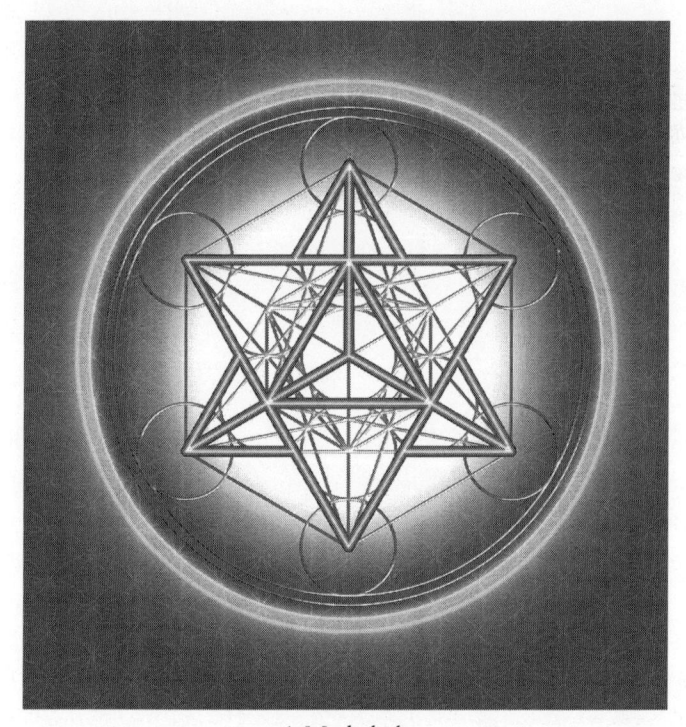

A Merkabah

The Merkabah is a metaphysical energy field that surrounds the human body made up of tetrahedrons (three-dimensional triangles) that rotate around the body. A slowly rotating Merkabah is considered not good, but that is the case or worse for many humans today. Worse, their Merkabah may have come to a hard stop. There is a specific meditation that, if done properly, can restore your Merkabah's rotation and allow for ascension to higher consciousness.

Almost a year later as I was speaking with a friend, she mentioned the Isis cards, and the conversation really connected all those dots that had been placed over the past year. Her suggestion to wear lapis lazuli, the Isis cards, and the Merkabah all came together in this one conversation. There was no way I could dismiss any of it this time. I immediately got the crystals, and the cards and did more research on the Merkabah.

That research led me to Maureen St. Germain, the much-respected founder of the Ascension Institute Mystery School Inc., near Sedona, Arizona, with branches Transformational Enterprises Inc. and Akashic Records International Inc. She has written *Waking up in 5D*, *Opening the Akashic Records*, and *Beyond the Flower of Life*.[8] *Beyond the Flower of Life* is the book I was guided to, and it started me on the path to connecting with my higher self and activating my Merkabah.

Closely connected is the term Ma'aseh Merkabah, meaning "The Account of the Chariot" or "The Works of the Divine Chariot" as told in the first chapter of Ezekiel and seen in early Jewish mysticism, c. 100 BCE–1000 CE, speaking of the heavenly palaces and the throne of God.

Maureen began her Merkabah journey with Drunvalo Melchizedek with a simple course at his Seed of Life Institute. Drunvalo was a lifelong researcher and lived among shamans and indigenous people throughout his research of ancient history and culture.

Maureen was one of the last students trained to teach the Merkabah meditation by Drunvalo before he closed his school. Though there are many critics of Drunvalo and no doubt Maureen St. Germain as well, I encourage you to follow your own intuition if you wish to investigate further.

Maureen recommends a forty-five-day period while you work daily at connecting with your higher self and learn to trust the information that you receive in this process. She recommends no other divination tools be used during the forty-five-day time frame.

I participated in the forty-five-day practice about a year ago but never gave up my Isis cards. Just under a month ago, I started those forty-five days over again with no divination tools. I now know to trust the answers I get when I ask my higher self a question, and I recognize the subtle answers are true answers from my higher self.

During this period, I also practiced my Merkabah meditation passed down by Maureen and still do daily as we speak. I originally did this meditation from her voice-recorded meditation and did see an improvement in my higher self-connection. This time around though, I purchased her four-hour instructional video, and it taught me a few things that I was doing wrong. If you are interested in learning this Merkabah meditation, I would certainly suggest reading the book *Beyond the Flower of Life* and then the four-hour training. It will be worth your time and money. The tools she provides have been huge in connecting with my higher self and helping me operate on a more holistic view of my world and the world around me.

I can honestly say that after my Reiki attunements, my Merkabah practice has been the most life-changing practice in my ascension journey. I have received so much emotional, spiritual, and physical growth in all areas of my world. I've become so much more present with my thoughts and actions, much more disciplined in my eating habits and physical activity, and pay so much more attention to my goals and how to get there.

I now trust that I have the ability to achieve any of the goals I set forth in my life. I know that I can obtain anything I can dream of the ability to overcome any obstacles that get in my way. I now know that I have the answers; I just need to listen and follow the signs.

I know that because you are here now, you've heard of the law of attraction. It would be nearly impossible for you to not have, given the subject matter and our time and place right now. The more I learn about the law of attraction, how we think, and how to control our thoughts and emotions, the more I love and truly enjoy the whole process of manifesting my dreams.

I recently attended a five-day manifestation challenge that corresponded with the new moon. I spent this time in gratitude for the amazing life I now have and the blessings that already exist in my everyday life. In my daily meditations, I followed up my Merkabah meditation with its usual unity meditation sending love out to the entire universe. This I followed up with some visualization of me on stage speaking to the audience at book signings around the world, sharing all the things I've learned with you so that you can find your own divine path of consciousness.

Repeatedly, I heard, "You've got to write the book. You've got to write the book." So I began writing again. At this time, I was about halfway through my first draft. I think it was day two of this challenge when I decided I needed to write every day and I started to do so. Each day, I make my list of the three most important things I need to get done that day: (1) write 2000 words, (2) read one chapter in my textbook, and (3) stay on plan with my meals and my exercise.

Every day if I get those things done, then I know I'm having a good day. If I continue to get those three things done, then I'm on my way to achieving my dreams. These three things will likely change over time, but making that list and getting it done each day is imperative to me and progress.

With the law of attraction, what we think about we bring about, so if I partake in inspired action every single day for each of my goals and dreams, then I am bringing myself one step closer to those dreams being real and present.

Part of managing our thoughts is noticing when we are focused on the negative side of our mindset. Our minds can take us on a wild ride if we let them, and I can't deny that mine still does now and then. Today though, I find I am getting better and better at noticing when I'm thinking more negatively in the moment versus the past version of me going days or maybe even weeks on a downward spiral.

Gratitude every single day is one of the things that keep me present, humble, and gracious. I am very aware of how lucky I am every single day, whether things are going according to plan or not. I know that I am blessed to have clean air and water, a wonderful marriage, a beautiful home, healthy and productive children, and a career that allows me to serve in a way that lights me up in body, mind, and spirit.

Each day during this manifestation challenge, I spent time going deep into visualizing what I really wanted as if it was real right then. In those meditative moments, I've visualized over and over again standing on stage with this book, speaking to you, and sharing all I've learned on my journey.

I've rehearsed the words I'd say over and over again. I've felt the excitement and the nerves. I've traveled to and from events and arrived home again, sharing it all with my husband over and over in my mind. I already know what this would feel like.

One day after I finished my manifestation challenge, I was on the couch watching *The Big Bang Theory*, and the phone rang. It was Balboa Press. I asked my higher self. Is it in my highest good to take this call? The answer was a clear yes.

I spoke with Rich, and he gave me all the details and options for self-publishing. I had chosen two different packages to discuss with my husband, and Rich would call me back on Monday evening. I later discussed it with John, and he decided he would attend the call on Monday evening.

I knew that we had recently had some big expenses, and this might not be in the cards right now, but I trusted that all would happen for my highest and best good and released it to the universe. At the same time, I was pretty sure John would approve the more expensive package, but we would have to wait and see.

Monday evening arrived, and John made it home in time for the meeting. I asked questions I knew he'd want to know, and in the end, he just nodded his head and gave me his card. A few minutes later, he got up and said, "Do you need me anymore?" and he went outside.

After the call, I followed him outside, beyond excited to say thank you. His reply was "How could I say no?" In all actuality, he could have said no, but he didn't and I am once again so grateful for another amazing blessing and manifestation and that my husband has faith in my dreams and is willing to invest in those dreams. I know this was manifested, and even though I had truly released the whole situation to the universe, I knew that we were going to end up where we did.

Last September, I had a similar experience. I had been taking some metaphysical classes, and one of them was on manifesting. I participated in a week of manifestation meditations. At that time, I was manifesting the fully loaded Range Rover that would take me to all my speaking engagements. I had no idea how I would do this and assumed it would be a more long-term manifestation.

The following weekend, we went up north to see the family. On our way home, we had just come off one highway onto another, and all of a sudden, there was a ton of fog. I thought, *Where did all this fog come from?* I heard a *beep, beep, beep* from the car and then a slam. I ran into the person in front of me. This pickup had a malfunction and spewed out a bunch of black smoke, so I couldn't see a thing. Luckily, no one was severely hurt, but our one-year-old car was totaled. I instantly knew it was toast.

At the same time, I was fully aware that we had been 100 percent protected in this accident. Thank you, angels. It wasn't until the following weekend when we purchased our new car that I realized that I had manifested this through the law of attraction and the practices that I'd been working with.

I did not get a Range Rover, but I did drive a couple and decided it wasn't all I thought it would be. But I did purchase a Nissan Rogue Platinum, and she is truly my baby. I love this car, and I'm looking forward to it taking me wherever I need to go with her for a very long time.

The longer I think and work in this manner, the easier it gets. It really does become second nature to think positively, in gratitude for the present moment, and believe that you can attain whatever your heart desires if it is aligned with your true self and for the highest good. I naturally just think of three things I'm grateful for first thing in the morning and last thing in the evening. This is the way I begin any prayer or meditation. Then I visualize the things I want to create in my life, and I always ask them to allow me to serve in a way that lights up my body, mind, and spirit.

For the past few days, I've been looking forward to my one-year review at work. I'd been manifesting a certain amount of a raise and a promotion. That promotion was rather vague in my mind as to what that looked like. This afternoon when I had my review, I did receive a very generous raise and a new opportunity that I am very excited to be of service to.

As I was visualizing this raise, I focused on the number 8. As discussed earlier, eight is my personality number and my life path number, so that was my focus. I did receive a good raise, it wasn't the one I had imagined, but it was very close.

10

FOOD TOOLS FOR HEALING

Let food be thy medicine and medicine be thy food.
—Hippocrates

Though I grew up in a fairly healthy home and my mom and dad were all about whole foods and raising their own foods, I really had no idea how important this was until I was diagnosed with Crohn's disease close to forty years old.

When my doctor suggested long-term steroids, I decided there had to be a better way. So I went home and started doing my research. I soon realized and still say this today: couponing gave me Crohn's. Let me explain. For the past few years, I had been doing the couponing game, clipping coupons, and getting the cheapest prices on the cheapest things I could fit into my single-mom-of-two budget.

If you've ever used coupons to any extent, then you already know that you usually can't buy anything of quality with a coupon. Coupons are most often only for overprocessed and packaged foods. These foods shouldn't even be considered foods, and that is exactly why I ended up where I did.

At a certain point, our body cannot recognize these things as food anymore. With my clients, I always use a Dorito as an example, but you'll get the drift. When we eat a Dorito, our body doesn't know what to do with it. While it's trying to decide, it will place those particles in fat cells while it does the more important work. Then our fat cells say, "I don't know what to do with this either," so they tense up and hold on to those particles and won't let them go because they don't know what it is.

Over time, this process clogs our fat cells and creates disease in our bodies. In my case, I had created a chronic inflammatory bowel and digestive tract, but I wasn't willing to live with this for the rest of my life. I was going to do something about it and not with steroid medications that I'd never be able to get off.

I began my research, looking for a natural way to relieve my pain and the anxiety that came along with such a disease. I bought book after book, read article after article, and watched video after video, just trying to find a solution.

In that search, I found food. Yes, food. Could it really be that simple? Yup, whole clean food. Not food in plastic and cans, but real food from the ground and the trees, food that was raised or grown in a clean and healthy way. It was all about the food.

When you look back in time, it has always been about the food, going back 3,000 years ago when Ayurveda was the common practice. Ayurveda is a natural system of medicine originating in India. Derived from the Sanskrit words *ayur* (life) and *veda* (science or knowledge), this was *the* science of life. Ayurveda was brought to the United States in the 1970s by the great Yogi Maharishi Mahesh when he also brought transcendental meditation on his journey to the States.

Today, Ayurveda is legally practiced in all fifty of the United States, yet many people have never even heard of it. Ayurveda is based on the idea that disease is due to imbalances or stress in a person's consciousness. It encourages certain lifestyle interventions and natural therapies to regain balance between the body, mind, and spirit.

The practice focuses on a range of treatments, including *panchakarma*, also referred to as the five actions. These actions are yoga, massage, acupuncture, and herbal medicine to encourage health and well-being.

It also has a great deal of focus on five elements, which are ether (*akash*), air (*vayu*), fire (*agni*), water (*jal/pas*), and earth (*prithvi*). They are the center of the Ayurvedic principles. They represent the fundamentals of nature and matter.

In Ayurveda, our characteristics are referred to as having certain properties. There are three in total and are called doshas. Those three are *vata*, *pitta*, and *kapha*. Each person will be more dominant in one or two of these properties than the other(s), but we are all a combination of all three. This just refers to your tendencies in general. Nothing is considered good or bad, just balanced or unbalanced.

Living an Ayurvedic lifestyle would revolve around the seven principles of psychic consciousness: thoughts, emotions, relationships, diet, daily rhythm, lifestyle, season, and environment. The whole of these seven principles is what influences the balance and imbalance of the above three doshas.

It's a very interesting practice and will pair food choices that will counteract the symptoms you are feeling with foods that are considered the opposite. This is one of the first things I explored while trying to figure out my healing process. To this day, I will fall back on a good old *kitchari* when I'm not feeling well. Kitchari is a porridge-like dish made with rice and dal (split peas) and is just very healing in general, no matter what your doshic constitution.

Though I don't live a strict Ayurvedic lifestyle, I fall back on its principles often. I do see a local Ayurvedic practitioner and have reached out for her advice from time to time as I maneuver my own journey to well-being.

In fact I just saw her yesterday for a beautiful fall glow massage with all her nurturing oils and herbs that just bring me to a beautiful place of balance. Ayurveda is not just about food. It is truly a holistic approach to well-being and essentially focuses on prevention versus reaction in our bodies and minds.

I did initially settle on a dietary theory called the specific carbohydrate diet, containing no gluten, no sugar, no processed foods, and only dairy with no lactose and specifically made. This diet was very helpful in my healing process, and I still feel blessed to this day that I found it when I did. As I dove into this new eating lifestyle, I felt better and started to lose weight. I had more days where I wasn't afraid to leave the house or that I'd lose my job because I was never at my desk and always in the restroom. I was starting to take my life back one bite at a time, one meal at a time.

There were still times when the flares were intense and emotionally draining. I remember calling an old friend whom I hadn't seen in years. He had become a holistic chiropractor. In tears, I begged for an appointment and some help. He fit me in the next day. Thank goodness.

When I got to his office, we went over all that was going on and what I was doing, and we began the exam. I was amazed when he agreed with most of my decisions about food, teas, and other things I'd started using. He prescribed a good probiotic and a few other supplements. I started on his plan immediately and literally felt improvements the next day. I continued to see him regularly until we moved in 2020. I will still give him a call to see if he can fit me in when I'm in the area. I've still never found a comparable doctor anywhere in my area.

This is an area that can give us great relief from our ailments if we are willing to take the time to learn and try new things. Back then, I ended up with SCD (a specific carbohydrate diet), but there are so many dietary theories out there that can be beneficial when it comes to healing your body. Everyone's body is different, and everyone's journey is different. My advice now is to always be your own advocate and find a medical or wellness professional who is truly on your side. There are options. We just need to be willing to explore them.

Unfortunately, this was not the end of my Crohn's flares by any means, but they were getting further and further apart and hung in there for less time every time they appeared. I kept digging to find answers. I'd come so far but still needed more help and had a long way to go.

I soon realized. It wasn't *all* about the food. I noticed that my flares would rear their ugly head not because I was eating badly (because I wasn't) but because my stress was out of control. My stress levels were triggering my flares.

This is where lifestyle comes into play. Managing our stress is so unbelievably important in managing our health. Stress is the cause of 90 percent of chronic illnesses, and it was certainly affecting mine.

I remember coming home one day and saying to my daughter, "I'm reading that I should meditate, but I don't know how." She, at fourteen, said, "Come on, Mom. It's easy. Go get this app." The app was Headspace and I loved it. I did a free trial and loved the Aussie accent of the little orange guy. It was so calming. I started meditating every day and, within a week, saw a difference in my stress level and how I moved through my days and nights. I just started to roll with things better and literally go with the flow. It was like I'd opened the door to this calmer world.

My flares happened less and less, and I was feeling better and better all the time. I continued to lose weight and heal my gut. This is when I decided to become a meditation instructor. I had to help others find this kind of peace in their lives. I've studied mindfulness, Ayurveda, and Ho'oponopono meditation and still can't get enough of it.

Two years ago, I moved to a more plant-based diet as I still had trouble digesting animal protein. I found that plant-based proteins worked much better for me and continued to work toward that kind of lifestyle. Now I am fully plant-based, and my digestion is better than ever and my Crohn's disease has been in remission for over a year. I feel amazing and in the best health of my life.

I've discovered other benefits to living plant-based as well. First, when I went plant-based, of course, I did what I do. I started doing more research on the subject. When I did, I discovered so many things about the treatment of animals, the cruelty that is out there, the state of our planet, and how a plant-based diet can help so much in all these areas. It brought my attention to several things that I had just discarded as not a big deal.

I know now that every one of my choices in life is important and I can make a difference in the world just by making decisions that align with my core beliefs. That being said, I am certainly not the perfect citizen and I'm sure there are things I could do better, but I do feel better about the decisions I have made when it comes to my food, the animals, the planet, and my health as a whole.

Changing over to a plant-based lifestyle has not only affected my weight-loss struggles and my digestive health but it has also opened up my spiritual pathways. I have a much clearer connection with my higher self, I can settle into much better and deeper meditative states, and my spiritual gifts are becoming crisper and clearer every day. The visions I see are clearer and more vibrant. The things I hear are more like voices than thoughts. That sense of knowing is undeniable when it shows up, and I can act in confidence on the information that I receive.

Each morning when I go to my crystals to see what I should carry with me that day, there is no doubt in my mind which one is best. When I ask my higher self a question, I rarely question the answer anymore. When I visualize something I want to manifest in my life, there is no doubt that it will be a part of my life. I know that it's already done and I will see it in time.

My physical body thanks me every day with less pain and inflammation, better movement and flexibility, and more energy to do all the things I used to think I did not have time to do. I've even added more things to my schedule than before.

On a normal weekday, I rise at 4:00 a.m. and head downstairs to the gym. When I'm done with my workout, I'll come back up and grab a cup of coffee, maybe set some intentions for the day (my top goals for the day), and at 5:00 a.m., I'll take the doggie for a walk. We'll return at 5:30 a.m., and I'll sit down for meditation, usually my Merkabah meditation followed by the unity breath. This morning after my meditation, I went to my sound room to record some meditations I've written. Sometimes depending on the time I have, I'll grab a full moon or new moon meditation or whatever else strikes me at the time. Then I'll hit the shower, gather my lunch, maybe do some dishes and the floors. I'll take a look at the menu for the night and get anything I need ready if I can. Then I'm off to work.

On my drive, my audiobook is always on. I'm always listening to something plant-based or health-related or a spiritual piece by a number of amazing authors like Wayne Dyer, Louise Hay, Gabrielle Bernstein, and many more. I am the audiobook queen.

During my lunch break, I'll write or create some meditations. This is one of those things I just love to do. On other days, I'll study some nutrition knowledge. I'm currently working on my sports nutrition certification. Still other days, the girls and I will get out and go for a walk.

Usually, the end of the day is a little less packed. I'm clearly a morning person, but I do often continue writing or studying after dinner, taking the dog out, and watering the garden. Once I sit down for dinner, not much else gets done. I used to feel guilty about not cleaning up the kitchen most nights, but now I forgive myself.

John has also found lots of benefits to his more plant-based lifestyle. He knows he feels so much better physically. He has less pain, and I don't think he's had a gout flare since he started his transition to a more plant-based life.

He has had a spot on his chest for years that always looked terrible. I've always been concerned about it. It used to be about the size of a quarter, and it was always red and flaky dry skin. It never seemed to go away. He consistently put frankincense on it, but it was always there. I'd been convinced it was cancer forever but, at some point, decided I was just bringing negative energy to it and let it go.

Last month, he came to me and said, "Check this out. Since I went plant-based, this thing has totally disappeared." He wasn't kidding. There is no sign of it at all. That thing has been there for over twenty years. Needless to say, I am thrilled, and even though he always thought I was nuts, I think he is too.

He came home the other day and said, "Did you hear the news? The FDA has approved meat made in a lab." I'd seen this in a documentary a few years back and they are taking stem cells from cows and growing burgers in a petri dish. Of course, leave it to our government to make this part of our food supply. John said right then and there, "I don't think I'll ever eat another piece of meat. That's disgusting." I tend to agree.

When talking about food in general and our health, there are so many dietary theories that can be helpful to people. The key is to do your research and listen to your body. Our bodies will tell us what we need to know. We just need to start listening.

That means when you eat an ice cream and fill up with phlegm or indigestion or have an asthma attack, your body is trying to tell you something. When you eat tomato sauce and get heartburn, your body is trying to tell you something: not that you should go get a Prilosec but that the tomato sauce doesn't agree with you. When you eat corn and you all of a sudden have joint pain, it's probably the corn and likely genetically modified corn. Corn, like soy, is very much genetically modified, especially in our country. Always buy both organic. Organic is non-GMO.

Part of the problem is that we have been ignoring our bodies for so long that we don't even notice anymore. We just know we never feel good because our bodies are always inflamed, and we don't know which thing or things are causing it. This is where an elimination diet comes in and can be so helpful if you are committed to seeing the light at the end of the tunnel.

With an elimination diet, we remove all those items that are likely causing inflammation in your body. These things are usually sugar, alcohol, gluten, and processed foods. Other programs remove well-known allergens like eggs, dairy, shellfish, gluten, etc. There are different time frames to do this, depending on the dietary theory you are abiding by but usually a minimum of six to eight weeks.

Then you start to add things back to your diet one thing at a time so you can notice what your body is reacting to. This way, you're starting with a clean slate and will notice if there is an issue. When I started the SCD (specific carbohydrate diet), I eliminated a lot of things. When you start this one, you start with a very limited variety of bland food but start to add things in a little bit at a time after a week or so.

The first week of any elimination diet is generally the toughest part. Many people experience some negative effects like tiredness, joint pain, muscle aches, headaches, and more. This is usually due to a detox period and/or what they call a die-off. When dealing with gut issues, die-off is quite literally the die-off of the bad bacteria in your gut. These beginning parts of these diets will quite simply starve out the bad bacteria in the gut that are causing the imbalance between the good and the bad in our body.

Our gut is basically the home front of our immune system. It is the home of 100 trillion different bacteria, both good and bad. The key is to keep the good and bad in a good balance. When the bad bacteria have a chance to get the upper hand, that is when the trouble begins. This can happen in several ways. The most common and well-known is repeated antibiotic use, but any interruption in the balance of the microbiota can be the cause. It can be the result of a dietary change such as increased protein, sugar, processed foods, or even pesticides.

Typical symptoms include gas, bloating, irritated bowel, heartburn, or even weight gain or loss. An occasional bout of one of these symptoms is not something to be concerned about, but if you experience these issues regularly, you might want to consult your doctor.

Some easy things you can do to help your situation may also help avoid medications or worse. First off, look at your diet. An elimination diet is a great option, but if it seems a little too intense, you can start just by cleaning it up a bit. Remove sugar and processed foods. That might be all you need to fix your problem. Pay attention to how your body reacts to the foods you eat. Even better, start to journal everything you eat. It might seem like a pain, but when you find out what's causing the problem, you'll be so glad you did. Take a quality probiotic. These are good bacteria in the gut. Drink lots of water. We all should be doing this every day anyway, but it certainly can help in this situation too. Take your time when you're eating. Make a point to chew your food well. At least twenty-five chews per bite of food is a good place to start. I know this sounds ridiculous, but once you start, you'll soon find yourself at fifty. This serves two purposes. One, you break down your food better in two ways, with your teeth and with your saliva, giving your gut less work to perform after the food is swallowed. Two, if you take longer to eat your food, your hunger monitoring system has time to stay in check and let you know you've had enough to eat. In turn, you don't end up with excess food in your gut that doesn't get fully digested and unfortunately sits and rots in the intestines.

Sleep is another super important part of any health regimen. When you sleep, your body does maintenance and repairs. If we're not getting seven to eight hours of sleep per night, our body doesn't have the time it needs to complete that maintenance process.

To add to the problem when we don't get our allotted amount of sleep, our cortisol levels will rise, which in turn slows our metabolism. Cortisol means stress, and stress means you're operating from your parasympathetic nervous system. So this means your body is in emergency mode and is not functioning optimally.

Finally, check your stress levels. If there's one thing I learned, it's that I can eat 100 percent right, but if my stress level is over the top, then my Crohn's symptoms will take over and there's nothing I can do about it.

Our gut is truly the home base for our health. Our immune system basically lives in our gut. Have you ever heard of the gut-brain connection? There is actually a two-way biochemical signal that takes place between the gastrointestinal tract and the central nervous system, also referred to as the gut microbiota. There are several techniques to reset the brain-gut, including progressive muscle relaxation, visualization, and restful music, all of which I am a big fan of and have used personally in the past and present. Research shows that these therapies are very effective, even more so when combined with cognitive behavioral therapies (CBT).

CBT is a psychosocial intervention that aims to reduce symptoms of various mental health conditions such as depression and anxiety. This may seem extreme, but if you've ever suffered from extreme digestive disorders, then you can likely understand this position. I know when I was in the depths of Crohn's disease, I was certainly suffering from some level of depression as well as anxiety. I was often living in fear of not being able to leave my own house for fear of finding the nearest restroom in time. These kinds of feelings can change a person's life in a drastic way in a very short period.

I find our diet is our first line of defense when it comes to any ailment in our bodies, but I also have found many other tools that can be added to a healthy diet to improve the overall lifestyle as well. Yoga and meditation are a couple of other areas that can assist both physically and emotionally.

Have you ever heard the saying "All disease begins in the gut"? This really is no joke. When we move to an anti-inflammatory diet that is devoid of harmful things like sugar, dairy, gluten, alcohol, and processed foods, our health starts to change almost instantaneously. Most people will see a visible difference in a matter of days and start to see significant changes in a two-week period.

11

MINDSET, MINDSET, MINDSET …

> Positive anything is better than negative nothing.
> —Elbert Hubbard

This morning when I got out of bed, I was dragging. I didn't want to get up. I didn't want to work out. I didn't want to go for a walk. I just didn't want to play today. But I did. I often don't want to get out of bed and often don't want to go work out when I open my eyes in the morning. That being said, I push myself to do exactly that five days per week. I have to because I know that the second I don't follow through with the things that are going to get me where I want to be, that's the second that I start *not* achieving my dreams.

This leads me back to the book *Kiss That Frog*. That book made so much sense to me, and it works so well for me that I try to live those principles every day. Yet this morning, I was feeling like I wasn't hitting my goals like I should be.

I got up at 4:55 a.m., went downstairs, drank water, poured coffee, and headed downstairs to do my workout (still not feeling it). I pushed my way through my core workout feeling a little bit in a fog. I was tired with a capital T.

When I finished up and headed back upstairs, I realized it was getting lighter a little later now, also a bit of a bummer in reality. So I decided to switch it up and do my meditation before taking Tobias for our walk. Maybe that would get me in the groove.

So I settled into my Merkabah meditation, the unity breath, and some gratitude practice until Tobias was nudging and fussing at me. Then off we went for our two-mile walk. My mind was going a hundred miles an hour, trying to figure out how to get out of this funk. As you can see, I hate it when my vibration is off.

All the possibilities ran through my mind as to why I was feeling this way this morning. Am I just too tired? Did I eat badly yesterday? Is it because I didn't accomplish all my top three goals yesterday? That must be it. I didn't write yesterday. But how was my food? Maybe this new macro plan is not what I need. Maybe it's too hard for my body to digest. Tobias, what the heck are you doing this morning? You're making me crazy. Can we just walk? What can I do to fix this mood? What the heck is wrong with me? How am I going to get all this stuff done today? I don't want to be in a lack mindset, but I need more time. No, I don't. It's all going to be fine. It went on and on and on.

I got to our turnaround point, and it was like flipping a switch. Oh my god, I just need to shut it down for a minute. I just need to stop the chatter, the noise.

Breathe, Candy. I started to breathe in through my nose. I imagined it sweeping away all those thoughts with each inhale. Then I'd breathe out through my mouth and let it go. I continued with this pattern until I thought, "This would be a good meditation to record … Oh right, here I go again. Breathe in through the nose, sweep up all that mind trash, and let it go with the exhalation." I noticed the sun rising and bringing some peace to it.

I started to feel a little better by the time I got home. I was able to let go of all the craziness going on in my head and just enjoy the rest of my walk, which is usually the best part of my day. I was able to enjoy the view and the peace on the way back home. My mood is still a little wonky today, but I'm not going to spend my whole day worrying about it. I'm acknowledging it and moving on with my day. It will change as I go.

I refuse to dwell on it and allow it to get worse and more intense. This is sometimes the key: to find that place of balance where you allow yourself to feel whatever emotions you are in at the time while not losing yourself in the drama that they have the ability to create for you. This too shall pass.

That is not a normal morning for me these days, so when I do feel in that funk, it can throw me for a loop because I rarely have those days in my life, but sometimes it's unavoidable. I believe if I dug into the astrology of today, I might find there is some sort of heavy energy lingering about us, but whether I know what it is or not, I still have to deal with it effectively.

This is the mindset that I have selected. This kind of thinking comes into play in so many areas of our lives. As this morning's scenario has just shown, I was able to use this to my advantage in more ways than one, just this morning.

My mindset when just getting out of bed this morning—it would have been so nice to just sleep in this morning, skip my workout and maybe even the walk, but that would not move me toward my goals, and it might even create a negative mindset tomorrow morning or even today.

I could have skipped my meditation as well this morning, but that wouldn't work in my favor. I know that my meditation improves my day every day. That is not something I ever consciously avoid. It just makes too much of a difference in how my day plays out. Another way that demonstrates the benefits of mindset in our daily lives.

Oftentimes our mindset is simply a choice. Literally taking the time to recognize that it exists is the first part, which sometimes we miss altogether. Choosing to change that mindset is the next step. I choose to not let a funky energy take me out emotionally and keep me down all day. Once I recognize it, give it a little analysis, and feel it, then I'm able to let it go by consciously choosing to release it.

This morning, I recognized that I was just letting my mind run away with my thoughts. Once recognized, it serves no purpose to allow that kind of energy to continue. Sometimes it takes more than one try to actually move on from it, but you truly can make that choice.

When I got to work this morning, I realized I was still hanging on to some of that energy and still feeling a bit of the fog. So I grabbed some peppermint essential oil and got my diffuser going in the office to create some focus and concentration. I'm now feeling much more alert, upbeat, and enjoying the day. I never did figure out what it was all about this morning, but I've moved on now and I always feel better in a higher vibration.

I find this to be an issue with clients a lot as well. While coaching a weight-loss program, I see this every day. Often clients want to lose weight but are not willing to make any of the changes necessary to meet that goal.

I've had more than one person break down in tears in my office because they just need a creamy coffee. Yet last week, they were in tears when the doctor told them they were prediabetic and had high markers for heart disease. I'm reminded every day that weight loss is not just about food. This is true in all areas of our lives.

Clearly, mindset is not always as simple as deciding to change it. Often there are other physical, emotional, or even spiritual issues at the source. Sometimes the option to make that choice is not something that is currently available to us. That doesn't mean it will always be that way. Sometimes we need to chip away at it.

Just recognizing these patterns is a great start on the road to change. Once we recognize our minds racing a hundred miles an hour for no apparent reason or even for some good reason, it gives us the opportunity to analyze and potentially make some changes, even if it's just to quiet those thoughts for a few minutes a day. That in itself can make a huge difference in one's life, one quieter moment at a time.

Meditation is my favorite way to get my emotions and my vibrations in check, but I also find that my daily workout does amazing things for my mind as well. In general, my self-care routine is pivotal to my well-being. That routine of getting up, working out, walking, and meditating gives me some quality time with myself to check in and provide some true self-care and grounding to start my day.

Whether we believe it or not, we all need self-care every day. Taking care of ourselves first should absolutely be a top priority. I know each day when I headed off to work to take care of all the other people that I encountered during the day, I came first and I was OK. That saying "You can't take care of anyone else until you take care of yourself" is god's honest truth.

So if this is a point of contention with you, then I suggest you take some time to try to change your mindset around this too. Taking care of me first is the number one best thing I've learned in my entire life. It must happen, and without that, I cannot thrive, I cannot help others, and I cannot be happy. I must take care of myself first.

We have the tools to change our mindset around anything. There used to be a time when I thought I was not worthy of wealth, a nice car, a job I loved, or even to write a book or claim to be a coach. I have changed my mindset around all these things, and now realize I can be anything I want to be and prosper in any area I wish to prosper. I just need to believe it and act on it.

The areas where we might want to begin when working on our mindset can start with letting go of some things like negative self-talk. I know we all know what this is and oftentimes don't even know we're doing it. This can be anything from making a mistake and saying to ourselves, "Well, that was stupid," or calling ourselves fat or making fat jokes about us. There's a million ways we've learned to berate ourselves.

Letting go of those limiting beliefs is a biggie and also one we may not even realize we have. Tell me, do you believe you can reach your goals and dreams? Is that possible? Or do you believe deep down that you will never get there? That you're not worthy, smart enough, small enough, pretty enough, or rich enough? The list goes on and on, and we may not even know why we feel this way.

Oftentimes we learned these beliefs from our parents, who passed them down to us. Maybe it's something someone said to you a long time ago. I just last year realized that my deep-seated belief that I was not smart enough came from a third-grade teacher who told my mom that I'd never be a good student and my belief that I could not manage money came from a combination of a failed marriage and those childhood beliefs.

These are things we don't even recognize doing as we work our way through our lives if we don't take the time to step back and analyze the patterns and actions of our journey. These are also things that can be of ancestral origin—thoughts, beliefs, and mindsets carried down from generation to generation.

I'm sure if you look close enough, you will find some limiting belief that has been carried down, shared, and taught from grandparents to parents to you and even to your own children. These are the wounds that take more work to heal than just one moment and decision, but it can be done.

Comparing ourselves to others is another one that we need to release ourselves from. While it's easy to want what others have, comparing yourself is like discarding everything you've got going for you at this moment. Admiration is great, as it's often a reflection of the great things we want for ourselves. Learn to distinguish between admiration and comparison and self-judgment.

Letting go of resistance is a huge way to change your mindset. If you want a different result, you need to do something differently. Making small changes consistently adds up and transforms your life. Though change is scary, we cannot expand and grow without stepping outside our comfort zone. To me, that feeling of discomfort means growth is happening.

Another biggie is letting go of our ego. I always think of Wayne Dyer when I hear this quote: "Would you rather be right, or would you rather be happy?" That one question really does say it all. Sometimes we just have to let it go.

Let's talk about what we should hold on to. The very first thing I think of when I want to change my vibe is gratitude. I know I've mentioned it before, but I truly believe that taking the time to think of three things I'm grateful for first thing in the morning and right before I close my eyes at night is one of the best practices I have. It can also be a good indicator of where my head is at that moment. I know that I have plenty to be grateful for every single day of my life. So if I can't think of anything when I start or end my day, then I *know* there is some work to be done.

The words "Just look around, there's always someone who's got it worse than you" are so true, and if I find myself not knowing what to be grateful for, that's a sign that I need to get a little humbler because my life is pretty blessed. I'm sure most of you can relate to that statement. Just the fact that I have clean water to drink and air to breathe is a lot more than many have.

Hold on to your energy and your purpose. It's important to make a conscious effort to carry yourself in a confident and purposeful way. Walk with pride by standing tall, and I guarantee you'll feel better almost immediately. Posture affects our mood, so we might as well soak up the benefits of it. Especially when we're feeling down and discouraged, stand tall and smile. It does change things.

Your energy is your energy. Don't let others come in and take that away from you. This can happen in several ways. Sometimes that is just one person coming into a room with a bad attitude and nothing good to say. Someone like this can be exhausting as well as robbing you of your own personal energy.

If you have people like this in your life on a regular basis, it might be wise to create some distance. Celebrate your own positive view on life and keep it close to your heart. Keeping a physical distance from these types of people can be a good idea too. Having someone in your physical space that is carrying this kind of energy can suck the life out of your aura. If you feel like they are too close and in your space, trust how you feel and create some physical distance between you. Protecting our energy at the start of the day can help too.

Purpose is a great one to hold on tight to. Purpose is that thing that lights us up and gives us energy. This looks different for everyone, and that is a good thing. It creates our individuality and makes us truly different from one another. What is it that lights you up, makes you happy, and puts a smile on your face?

This doesn't have to be just one thing either. I love to meditate and show others how to meditate. I love to help others feel better. I love to cook, create, and garden. All these things truly light me up and make me feel good. They give me energy and make me smile.

Usually when you're doing that thing you love, you're also surrounding yourself with uplifting people. That's because they are doing the same thing you are, and it makes them feel happy too.

Finding your purpose is easier than you may think. Many people make this a lot harder than it is. I feel that your purpose should be anything that makes you happy and allows you to help someone else while you're doing it. That doesn't have to be something that is a crazy obvious version of helping someone, like volunteering at a soup kitchen or handing someone cash. It can be as simple as singing a beautiful song. If you bring joy to other people with your song and that makes you feel good, that might be your purpose.

My purpose is to help other people feel better in their body, mind, and spirit. That shows up in several different ways. These ways vary from writing this book, writing a cookbook, creating meditations, or coaching someone on their wellness journey. These are all things that light me up and make me feel like I'm contributing to this world in a good way.

Surrounding yourself with uplifting people is another way to improve your mindset. Positive people love positive people. Negative people generally love to be negative, and they don't usually care whom they are negative with. I love being around people who are ambitious, creative, and inspirational to me to keep working hard and aiming for my life goals. Having someone negative around me all the time doesn't help me stay inspired and motivated to do the work I know I need to do to get where I want to be.

Give yourself some quiet time. A little time to yourself is a much-needed thing. We all need some of this, and even if we are uncomfortable with it, it's still important for us to do it. Allow yourself to get to know, like, and even love yourself. We spend our entire lives with ourselves. Don't you think it will be a much better ride if you enjoy who you're with 100 percent of the time?

Benevolence is another thing that can put a positive spin on your mindset. Doing something nice for someone else makes you feel so good, and it doesn't have to be something big. Last year on Christmas day, I went to my daughters for Christmas brunch. John and I had taken different vehicles because we were dividing and conquering the family responsibilities. I headed home and stopped at a gas station about halfway home to grab a coffee.

When I got to the counter, this girl was so cheery and helpful but in this store all by herself on Christmas Day. I grabbed a scratch ticket with my coffee and before I headed out the door, I pushed it her way, and said, "Merry Christmas." She looked totally shocked and said, "Oh my god, thank you so much." I smiled and went to my car. As I drove down the highway, I couldn't stop smiling as I was thinking, *I hope she wins a bunch of money*. Wouldn't that be cool? Of course, I'll never know, but that one little deed changed the whole energy of the rest of my ride home.

All these things we're talking about here are forms of self-care. That in the end is what it is all about. If we take care of ourselves first, then we have the energy to take care of all the other stuff that happens in our lives. Self-care gives us vitality, energy, and excitement to continue doing what we do every day. It can also inspire us to do something different and make some changes for the better.

Ironically, as I finish up this chapter on July 24, I look at some information I pulled for clients at the beginning of the month. This information is to bring their attention to the fact that today is International Self-Care Day.

This day was chosen for a reason, to remind us that self-care is needed 24/7 (pretty cute, ha).

The average person sees their doctor three times per year for about ten minutes, which leaves the rest of the time essentially self-care. That's pretty significant. Clearly, this is not just a buzzword or phrase. This is real and a huge part of our lives, which we need to give a little more attention to.

We need to stop ignoring our bodies and our minds and start taking better care of them every single day. It's a much bigger part of our overall wellness than our doctor even begins to play in our health.

Self-care includes all the things we do to maintain good health. That means good hygiene, eating well and healthfully, being physically active, being self-aware and conscious as opposed to self-conscious. It also means educating ourselves on important health topics, being proactive as opposed to reactive when it comes to our health, and finally utilizing the services available to us. This big picture looks different for each and every one of us and will most likely change over time. As we evolve as human beings and spirits, so too may our practices, interests, passions, and physical and emotional needs.

When thinking about self-care, be sure to take a holistic view. Include physical, spiritual, mental, and social aspects. When assessing the physical side, you might want to try a new activity or sport, start getting up and stretching or walking during your day, and incorporate a regular exercise routine. Don't forget about sleep; seven to nine hours per night is best. Of course, we can't forget our eating habits. Spiritually, we might give some attention to mindfulness practice, some breath work, time in nature, and positive self-talk, and we can't forget that we need vacation and adventure in our lives as well. Mentally, we can start with having self-compassion and knowing our limits. Expressing ourselves is very important for our inner truth. Start a new journey in anything that interests you. Allow yourself to enjoy hobbies and passions. That can lead you anywhere from reading a book to writing a book, looking at art, or creating art. Never count yourself as not capable or talented in any area that interests you. Socially, we can feel amazing by volunteering in our community, spending time with family and friends, and being there for others. If we don't have the time to spare, we can donate to charities that we are passionate about.

And let's not forget that we can enjoy this time too. Join a club or a group that brings you joy. That's what it's all about, right?

In all reality, mindset is a big part of our self-care, so staying in check with where your mindset is at is super important to remaining in flow with your life as you endure the ebbs and flows of this journey. We all know it's not all unicorns and rainbows, but the more present we are with our thoughts, the easier we will rise and fall with those ebbs and flows as we move through our lives with better grace and ease.

Take some time now to just analyze where you are in your daily mindset. Are you being supported by your current thoughts and actions? Or are those thoughts holding you back in your progress, your ambitions, and your accomplishments?

You have the ability to control the thoughts that go through your mind. Allow yourself the power to eliminate the poisonous thoughts and emphasize the ones that make you excited, stronger, and unstoppable. You can be all these things with a change of mindset.

12

FOLLOW WHAT YOU LOVE

*Passion is energy. Feel the power that comes
from focusing on what excites you.*

—Oprah Winfrey

Logic versus Passion

For much of my adult life, I operated on the logical end of the pendulum. When I was in high school, I intended to go off to college for art. I didn't have a plan beyond that at all. I just loved art. I loved painting, drawing, sculpting, and just creating any way I could with any materials I could get my hands on.

I know we've already discussed what happened from there. I didn't go to college, art school, or even hairdressing school. It was safer to not leave this little country town and do what the past three generations have done. Get a job and stay there, doing what we did, what we've always done. Success takes hard work. That would be too much fun. This was logical.

So I did. I took the first full-time job that gave me a paycheck because I was about to graduate and would be paying my parents' rent within a month. That job was hand sanding oak mirrors in a furniture factory. My reasoning was that my dad was a carpenter as were both of my grandfathers. One owned a business, and the other worked in a furniture factory. I'd be made for this.

I wasn't. It was awful. I would wake up every night sitting up in bed like I was sanding those mirrors. My hands were purple all the time from the oak. I hated the atmosphere. I hated the fact that you went on break when the bell rang, went back to work when it rang again, and went home when the bell rang again. It was the most robotic job I've ever possessed.

Then I went into retail—stocking shelves, folding clothes over and over again, and helping customers. This made sense; my mom owned a health food store, and I'd worked there for her before. I enjoyed this, but still, I had no goals and no future there. From there, I went to a health club as a front desk clerk. I loved the environment. I loved anything wellness, but It hadn't dawned on me that this might be a career-path opportunity. Maybe that was one of the universe's attempts to bring me into the wellness arena, and I just wasn't seeing it yet.

That job schedule was a little crazy, and I passed through a couple of office jobs here and there. Then I went to a retail catalog and had an office job there too. I was there for twenty-seven years before I was laid off.

During those twenty-seven years though, my health brought me back to the wellness arena again. This is when I became a health coach. I can't help but think the universe must have thought, *What the heck is this girl doing?* I had gotten my certification as a health coach but, at the same time, became an enrolled agent to do taxes.

I worked forty-plus hours, did some coaching, a lot of bookkeeping, and a lot of taxes. It wasn't long before I realized I hated doing taxes. I wasn't confident with what I was doing. Anytime anyone asked me questions, I assumed I'd screwed up. What made me think this would be my calling? It made sense. I was already doing bookkeeping, so it was only logical.

Just like it made sense twenty-seven years earlier to take the office job as it did to stay twenty-seven years. It was safe. It was logical. It wasn't frivolous, creative, or adventurous in any way. It was safe. The day I was laid off, I certainly didn't feel safe. I'm assuming that was the point. We can't play it safe forever and reach any of those big goals and dreams.

When I moved in with my current husband, that was one thing I made note of very quickly. He doesn't play it safe. He's all about taking a chance and putting himself out there. This, I see now, was the difference in how we were raised and what each of us saw every day growing up. My dad was a carpenter. He did work for himself, but his business never grew. He was happy in this little town of fifteen hundred people. My mom prided herself on bookwork (which must be where the logical part came from for me). They were content and happy. I'm sure they had their own goals and fears and uncomfortable moments and decisions over the years. I just wasn't seeing them.

John's family owned a large business that flourished for many years. He had his own logging equipment as soon as he turned eighteen. When that business closed, he left and became a business partner of another company. It seemed to me like he had no fear of failure.

What I didn't know is he did have the fear, but the need to be his own boss outweighed the fear of failure. Everyone's story is different, as are the challenges we all face along that path. Not everyone wants to be a big business owner. All of our passions are different.

When I started my own health coaching business, it was safe because I still had my full-time job. I also had the other bookkeeping jobs on the side and of course the coaching jobs on the side of that. When I look back now, I wonder. If I had stepped into my own power back then, would I have done an even better job by not stretching myself so thin? Would I have succeeded if I'd put my whole heart and soul into it? I guess we'll never know, but I can bet that if I had the mindset I do now, I would have made it with no problem.

Now there is no failure. Why? Because I'm acting out of passion instead of logic. I'm succeeding because I love what I do every day. I help people feel better every day. How can that be failing in any way at all? Yes, I still have dreams and goals—big goals. But I love my life at this very moment, and I am OK with where I am right now. The rest will come because I know it will. I can see it, I can feel it, and I can smell it. I'm creating it.

If you're still feeling fearful to jump right in the deep end, know that you're not the first and certainly won't be the last.

When I started as a health coach on my own, I began creating a cookbook. I was starting with baby steps, one recipe at a time. Before I knew it, I had over one hundred recipes. Then I self-published. This was so cool to me, more than I'd ever imagined. When we moved, I decided that I would become a personal chef and teach people to cook in their own homes and cook for personal parties in the evenings. I loved this until COVID-19 shut down the country and the world. That dream never came back, but I know that I reach so many more people every day than I could have ever dreamed of back then.

Today I love what I do. I can reach so many people and assist them in attaining better overall health. At the same time, I can record meditations for Insight Timer and write a book on the side as well. These are all little baby steps that can lead me to an even bigger and more rewarding career.

Can you imagine your dreams? That right there is really what it's all about. If you can imagine it, you can attain it. There's no doubt in my mind. That is why our God gave us an imagination.

So if you feel you're not doing what you really want to do. You're stuck in a job that you hate or just doesn't give you any joy? Take some time right now to imagine doing something you love. What is the first thing that comes to mind that you'd love to do?

Imagine that being your job, your partner, your home, your whatever. Allow it to play out in your mind how it would feel to live with this every day in your life. Keep it rolling. Allow it to grow in your imagination. The bigger the better. There are no limits to what we can do. If you can imagine it and you want it, then why can't you do it? God didn't put us on this earth to be mediocre. We were put here to be amazing and make our creator proud.

If you run into feelings of unworthiness, then think of your children. You wouldn't want your children to feel unworthy. You would want them to reach for the stars and create a better life than you've been able to create, right? The universe feels the same way. We are meant to be amazing and successful and do so with something and someone we love.

So allow your imagination to run wild. Create visions of your success. Create feelings of happiness and contentment. Imagine coming home each day feeling proud of all you accomplished in your job. There is no dream too large or too small. Whether a small-town carpenter with a hobby farm that lights you up or a big business owner leading your industry, it's your dream. You make it.

If you're not quite ready for this kind of activity, maybe just sit down with a piece of paper and write down the things you are passionate about. How can you invite more of these things into your life? Once you figure that out, take one action step to do it. This is inspired action.

Once I became a meditation instructor, I was so passionate about it. I to this day feel like everyone needs meditation in their life. I tried giving meditation classes for a couple of years and would have one person show up each week. I didn't make any money doing it because I had to pay for the space, but it was worth it to me to help someone alleviate their stress at the time. During the COVID shutdown, I did free live meditations on Facebook and had a lot of people attend. It made me happy and also kept me sane during that period of my life. It gave me purpose.

Now I create meditations weekly on Insight Timer and enjoy every moment of it. I love the whole process. I think of meditations at the strangest times, and I'm always amazed when these things come to me. Sometimes, I do a spur-of-the-moment channeled meditation too. That's the joy of it. It's spontaneous and fun, and people love it. I love recording them, editing them, and bringing them all together. I also love interacting with my followers after the fact. This simple little thing brings me such joy, not to mention the peace that comes with it.

Though most of us were raised to do the logical thing, especially when we're talking about our careers, I find logic is not always the best choice. I've gone the logical route. I will say I only had a few jobs that I truly didn't like, but now that I have one that I truly love, there is no comparison.

I think of my daughter when I talk about this subject. As she's finished art school, I am so proud of her. I do know though that she has dealt with so many people telling her along the way that she needs to get her head out of the clouds and get a real job, a real career, or a real life. I'll be honest, along the way, I may have done a little of that when she didn't make decisions that I thought she should be making.

Today she has a degree in textiles, and she is very passionate about it. That's the thing about passion. To me, I don't get it. Fabric is fabric, but to her, it is not. To her, there are companies who create great products with great fabrics and there are others who create expensive products with low-end fabrics, and this makes her mad. I love to see her in her element.

My oldest has lived passionately since she was a child. She's always held a strong opinion about most things, but when it comes to the things she's passionate about, that is hands down where she shines her light. She has always been a fighter, but she's also always taken care of what she needs first. She inspires me daily. I have learned so much from both. They each bring their own special and vibrant light to this world, and that is one of my biggest dreams come true.

Don't let others' opinions of what you are passionate about get you down or get in your way. Who knows, *your* ideas may be the next best thing that no one else has ever imagined. That's why we all have different views on life and in different areas of life. We're meant to be different and create new ideas every day.

There are many reasons to consider doing something you love for a living versus doing what may have always made sense. Money does not always conquer all when it comes to a career. Many people will choose a career that pays substantially less to do something that they're passionate about versus the logical choice.

A feeling of fulfillment at the end of the day can certainly go a long way. When I was sanding mirrors every day, I was not feeling fulfilled. My grandfather, on the other hand, probably would have felt a great sense of satisfaction at the end of each day because he'd created a beautiful piece of furniture for the world.

My fulfillment comes from helping people feel better in their bodies, their minds, and in spirit. My grandfather took great pride in his creations. My daughter takes great pride in being a part of a quality piece of clothing or home goods, by being sure the materials are of top quality. My other daughter is passionate about teaching children how important it is to take good care of their teeth. We all have a different idea of what a great job may look like, but that's what makes the world go round. We are all different, and we all love something different.

Your career should be more than just a job and a paycheck. If it's not, then I hope there is somewhere else in your life that fires you up. Your career should make you feel good emotionally, whether you are in or out of the office.

A job that you love will give you extra motivation to meet your goals, and when you do, a sense of accomplishment is amazing. It will make you more productive too. Now to me, *that* is logical. Of course, you're more productive when you love what you're doing. That makes total sense. If you are passionate about your job, you are likely to take an active interest in learning every aspect of that job, business, or industry. This is not only what sets you on a path toward success, but it also helps you get through the daily grind.

You will also be an inspiration to others. Too many of us are under the impression that you cannot have a job you love because you must work hard to earn money—that a job means hard and arduous work. It doesn't have to be that way.

There are lots of amazing and inspiring jobs in this world, and someone needs to do them. Why not you? Seriously, why not you? What makes you not worthy of enjoying your work every single day? This is usually a *big* question, and most people never seriously ask themselves this question.

When you really take the time to ask and think about this question, it may seem a little ridiculous as to why you've thought the way you've thought. Some people are afraid to follow their dreams of doing what they may love. I was. Why is that? Usually, it's because we don't want to step out and then fail. That's the thing though. If we never try, we'll never know if we'll succeed or not. So we've failed before we even began.

Others are afraid they'll succeed. Yes, afraid to succeed. I know it sounds ridiculous, but it's true for more people than you may think. Fear of success is a concern that once we achieve something new, we'll be incapable of sustaining it or may suffer because of it. Most people are not consciously aware of this fear. That's because when we focus on a goal, we talk about the positive outcomes of achieving the goal. Rarely do we share with others what might happen when we get there.

If you're at a place where you still don't know what it is you want to do for your career, your purpose, or your goals in life, I would pass along the tips that helped me find my place. First, think back to when you were a child. What did you want to do then? What did you want to be when you grew up? I didn't do this until I was forty-five years old. Up until that point, I was playing the logical game, and in reality, it really wasn't feeling logical at all.

Next, reach out to friends and family. Ask them what they think your strengths are. Oftentimes, those around us have a very different view of what we are all about, and when we are able to see things from the outside looking in, the light sometimes comes on.

Who was your role model growing up? This might seem silly, but I'll bet money that once you go down this road, some things may start to make you feel more in the true energy of you. Why did you love this person? This can uncover some deep intuitive stuff that you may have buried long ago.

Who knows why? Because someone criticized, commented, or laughed. Who knows? Do they have similar abilities, hobbies, and talents as you?

Finally, take some time to think about what you truly dislike doing. What are your core values, and where are these areas in which you don't want to make compromises? In my logical years, I always said, "I can do pretty much any job." And for the most part, that was not untrue. Then one day during those COVID days, I took a job working from home for a large lawn care company. This was work I'd pretty much done all my adult life, working in an office, on the phone and computer all day, and dealing with customers.

Yes, I could totally do this. The problem arose when I found out that the company was all about using horrible chemicals that aren't good for our planet, the people, or the animals. The more I worked there, the more I realized the moral code of the majority of people that I came in contact with was just not the same as mine.

I had too many calls with clients that said they'd canceled their programs six months ago and now someone was spraying their just-seeded lawn. They had watched employees pull in and park in their drive, sit on their phones for ten minutes, and then get out and stick a sign in the yard even though they hadn't done anything. I'd passed these complaints up the line several times to see them go nowhere. And the only solution was always "save the account."

I just couldn't do it anymore. So I quit. That was the only job in my life where I quit on the spot and didn't give any notice. It just was not a good fit for me at all. Paying attention to our moral compass is a super-important place to start when it comes to choosing a career.

When you feel deep in your soul that a position is not a good fit for you, listen to that intuitive information. We get these intuitive feeds for a reason. The day I planned to quit this job, I decided to work my shift and then I would be done.

Well, the universe had a different plan. When I picked up my first call that day, I had an angry client screaming at me again. As I went to get into his account, my computer went down. I struggled through that as my manager was telling me to save the account, and by the way, I did not. I picked up the next call, which was like a carbon copy of the last. Again, my computer went down. Once again, my manager was chatting with me to save the account. I replied, "Nope, and this is my last call. I will call you when I'm done here, so don't put any more through because I won't be answering them."

The universe was clearly telling me I did not belong here, so I took the hint, and I was done. If we don't listen, that higher power will scream at us if it needs to. Sometimes, we work hard not to hear what's being yelled from the mountaintops.

It is so important to listen and notice the things the universe is sending our way. Take some time to notice those things that you would normally just call a coincidence. Note how often those synchronicities happen. When a certain subject, job, career, or whatever comes up repeatedly. Someone might be trying to tell you something.

Being happy at work and loving what you do is an overall productivity booster and enhances performance. People who enjoy their jobs are more likely to be optimistic and motivated, learn faster, make fewer mistakes, and make better business decisions.

Finding work that interests and challenges you is an important part of loving your job. When you do the same tasks day after day, you may feel like you are ready for something new. When you get a variety of tasks and responsibilities that teach you something new, you may feel more engaged and fulfilled.

Sixty-five percent of US workers are happy with their jobs. But only 20 percent are passionate about their jobs. Likewise, only 49 percent of American workers report being "very satisfied with their work," while 30 percent are merely "somewhat satisfied." Over one hundred million US workers are at least somewhat satisfied with their work. I think we have a long way to go.

It's perfectly normal to love your job and, at the same time, recognize that it's hard work. Give yourself grace and balance when times get tough—but if you love your job, remember to be thankful that you do.

I truly love my job and feel very blessed to do what I do every day. I do have days though when I am exhausted at the end of the day, frustrated when I can't get through to people, or don't have the time to do what I want to do, but this is part of any job.

If you don't love your job, dread going in or even getting out of bed in the morning every single day, then you might want to take another look at the situation. Maybe it's time to let go of the sensible, logical, or reasonable side of things and start to dream a little bit. Take some time to think about what you would love to do if there were no limitations. Those are the things we are meant to create and birth into the world. Those are the things the world needs and is looking for.

When you use Google to look up the word *passion*, you'll get "strong and barely controllable emotion." That is where we want to begin when we think about what lights us up. Does it raise that kind of feeling within you? Strong and barely controllable? That sounds exciting to me, and that is when the real work gets done. That is where amazing ideas and discoveries come from. That is where dreams are made.

That is how it's supposed to be because that's the kind of emotion we need when times get tough and we need to keep pushing, grinding, and working through whatever comes up. That is the kind of emotion we need to keep creating, moving beyond the barriers that pop up and trying to stop our dreams. That is what it takes to not give up on the worst days and keep us moving forward, toward the great days when we are so grateful that we took the plunge and stepped out of our comfort zone just to do something we were passionate about and no longer could ignore that voice within us telling us to do it. Just do it.

Are you ready to take that plunge? Good, then make one move right now to start the process. I don't care what it is. Just take one massive step of inspired action to begin something you've been dreaming about and thinking about. Take one step to take this dream out of the cave that you've been hiding it in and release it to the world. The world needs it, and you need it.

13

HOW LONG DO WE IGNORE WHO WE REALLY ARE?

> Just be yourself. Let people see the real, imperfect, flawed, quirky, weird, beautiful, magical person that you are.
>
> —Mandy Hale

When we are children, we instinctively follow what we love. We don't give it a second thought when we're playing or talking or doing anything. As we grow older, we learn the rules of life, the rules that are taught to us by our elders and those who have been approved as our teachers. That is not to give teachers a negative annotation by any means. Please don't take this the wrong way. I am thankful to many teachers of mine over the years, and I think we all have one that comes to mind as making big contributions to who we are today.

My point here though is that we initially know what we love and naturally gravitate to that when we are born and are young. But as we progress in our society and become more a part of that society, we also become more of what society wants us to become. It is important to find ourselves again once we get there.

As I look around me and see those who have always marched to the beat of their own drum, I feel so much love for their sense of freedom and individuality. Our society may deem them weird, strange, or pretentious, but they are in touch with their true selves, and this is a feat. We all need to come back to our true creative selves. And when I say creative, I don't necessarily mean artistic, but that self that can create a life that is only true for you—that life that only you can imagine and create as only it should be for you. We are all individuals, and we are all different. Therefore, our life paths should all be different.

When I was a child, I honestly don't remember what I wanted to be. I do remember wanting to be an artist as I got older. I was good at it too. Then I started down my logical path, and we continued from there. At one time, I thought I'd lost myself because I didn't do anything in the creative realm anymore. I still don't do the art that I used to do, but I feel better about it now. I'm still creative in other ways, and I do hope to get back to the times when I could sit down and paint or draw. It will come.

Today my creativity is channeled into my writing, and I know that this is where it should be at this time. I have a message to share, and that is where I am guided to be and show my true self to the world.

How are you guided to share who you are? In some way, we are all here to help on some level, help others around us in some way. What is that for you? You may not even think you are helping anyone doing what comes naturally for you. I'm sure you are though, if you just think about it.

So many go through life without finding their true self. So many continue to follow the logical path and never find that thing that lights them up. So many continue on the journey of logic even though they despise it every day they open their eyes, drag themselves out of bed, and dread the journey to that job. No matter what it is, if it doesn't bring you joy if you dread it repeatedly every single morning. It's time to make a change.

But so many are stuck in fear, fear of what will happen, won't happen, or might happen. So stuck in fear that they can't take a step out of their comfort zone of misery. When you think about it, it really makes no sense at all. We're more comfortable staying in our own misery than we are stepping into what it is we love and are passionate about.

I say this because it was me. I stayed in that mediocre job for twenty-seven years before they laid me off. Thank God, they laid me off. Thank you, universe, for that intervention. I know now that the universe gave me so many chances to step out and do what I wanted to do, but I was too scared. I did dip one toe in the water, but I never really took the plunge, even after my layoff.

I was laid off in January of 2019. I had a six-month severance, which was a blessing. Yes, my mother-in-law got sick, and I had to help her. I counted that as a blessing that I was able to be there for her at that time, but did I use that as an excuse? Now I think I may have—an excuse not to go fully in.

In 2020 we moved, and the country shut down. I was trying to make my coaching business a success, but I had no faith in myself and even though I thought I was all in, now I see I really wasn't. I still had that intense fear of failure. I was still stuck in fear. I was still sitting in all those negative stories of my history, those things that had been said to me by teachers and an ex-husband. Those negative thoughts were still in the back of my mind.

So just how long do we ignore that true self within us? How long do we play it safe and spin our wheels in the mud of mediocrity? What is the thing that can and will pull us out of the sludge of life so that we can shine our own individual light proudly and confidently? This is what we are all meant to do and be. We are each meant to be a lighthouse in our own way.

I believe we find ourselves one piece at a time. I know I did. It's probably a good thing it happens that way. We might freak ourselves out otherwise. When I think about my journey, I'm pretty sure if it all happened at once, I would have been pretty freaked out.

I am truly a different person than I was one year, five, ten, and especially twenty years ago. I often remember the day when my husband said to me, "I can't wait to see what you blossom into." I still wonder if this is what he thought it might be. I'm fairly positive it was not.

Yes, we continue to be a great team, no matter how much both of us have changed over the past twenty-plus years. We are still each other's best friend and each other's rock. That in itself can be a huge help in finding yourself. When you know that your partner has your back no matter what, you can trust a lot more. It gives me a deeper inner strength, persistence, and focus.

We all have to have a rock to lean on, but it doesn't have to be a life partner or even a person. It can be in whatever form that is for you. And I hope you have both: someone here on earth *and* something bigger than that. No matter what your faith or belief system is, my recommendation is to immerse yourself in it. Feel the passion of your beliefs and continue to learn more about them and nurture them. Your spiritual base can carry you through some dark times.

All the tools in this book are a result of my exploring, learning, and growing into my faith and my belief system. That belief system, I know, is like no one else's, but I think that is how it's meant to be for all of us.

Finding my faith has been a huge part of finding myself. The process has been gradual and a bit piecemeal for me, but I've received so much from it as it has come to me. That something bigger than us is what shines the light on who we are really meant to be. That larger-than-life power can help us overcome all those fears that have been weighing us down and holding us back from bringing our dreams into reality.

Our fears keep us stuck. How long do we allow them to keep us stuck? How long do we keep up this charade, living a life of lack and unfulfilled dreams? When do we step into our power and take those first steps? Who will help you do that? Who will help you take that first step?

Though ultimately the power is within, we all need someone or something to back us up. Who or what is that for you? Where does your strength come from? Take some time to figure this out. I believe meditation was my first step in this direction. The day I started meditating was the day I started putting some faith in something bigger than me. That was the day I started allowing myself to think for myself and explore the possibilities.

I just had to stop the chatter in my mind. I had to quit the stuff that had been fed to me all my life, the stuff that I thought I had to or was supposed to do, how I was supposed to do it, and why I couldn't do it. That was my most limiting thing: the deep-seated belief that I wasn't worth or even capable of creating these dreams. So I didn't give them the time of day because what was the point?

I would wish things were different, but I wouldn't spend time dreaming about what I wanted. I spent a lot of time wishing it wasn't the way it was. Wishing my husband would behave differently, treat me better, or even be someone else. I would wish I didn't have so many bills, wish I had more money, wish I weren't so fat.

Yet I wasn't doing anything about any of it. I was enabling my husband to be who he was and allowing him to not treat me well. I was spending money I didn't have and then wishing I didn't have the bills. I was continuing to eat food that didn't serve my body, eat too much of it, and not move my body either, yet I was still wishing I wasn't overweight.

Meditation helped me quiet all the negative so that I could hear some tiny little pieces of the positive bit by bit, so I started to incorporate some new practices and some new thought patterns one little bit at a time. One positive thought would lead to another and another and another.

This is how you can do it too. Give yourself some time to just have quiet—quiet time from the people and activities around you, quiet time from your thoughts. Give yourself time to listen to your inner self and hear what it is that you want to be, how you want to feel, and what you want your life to look like.

Give yourself some time to let go of all those negative thoughts and start to latch on to some of the positive ones. From there, you will be amazed at the changes that will take place. The positive starts to outweigh the negative and you notice the negative much more than you used to. Then you realize that you hate the way you feel when you are in the negative, and you must change it.

This is when you are starting to take back your power and realize that you are the master of your mind and the thoughts that we keep in our minds are what we can create in our lives, and this is where the seeds are planted for our dreams. We are the creators of our own reality. Can you believe this? Even if you can't, give it a try and see what happens.

Give yourself five or ten minutes. I can tell you now it won't be easy the first time. I can hear you now telling me, "I can't stop thinking." I know. But we're not trying to stop thinking. We just try to quiet the noise a little for a while, acknowledging those thoughts and letting them pass. That will start to slow those thoughts, and eventually, you will find that space of peace. You will feel it in your body and in your mind, and you will want to do more of it. Try it.

If you have time right now, find a quiet place where you can go and not be disturbed. Take ten minutes to yourself. If you can't do it now, decide when you can take ten minutes for yourself today. Commit to it and do it today. Stop procrastinating and take that very first action step for you.

Sit somewhere comfortably and set a timer. I like to turn on "do not disturb" on my phone and set a timer for it. You will know your time is up when you start getting notifications again.

Sit comfortably up straight. Close your eyes, take a deep breath in, and then release it. Do these two more times, breathing in deeply and releasing fully. Then settle into a softer, more normal breath yet following it in and out of your body. As thoughts come into your mind, just noticing them is your priority here. Acknowledge them and then let them pass by.

Visualize them floating by like leaves in the wind or floating downstream, however, that vision may arise for you. Then come back to the breath. There is nothing else you need to do during this practice but that. Notice the thoughts, let them pass, and come back to the breath, mentally following it in and out. When the next thought comes up, do it all over again. This is the purpose of this practice.

When your time is up, take a moment to see how you feel. If some information came up for you, that's great, but that is not the purpose of this time. I encourage you to do this every day for a week and see what comes up in your life for you.

This will accomplish a couple of things. Number one, it allows you to take some time for yourself, a little bit of time that probably won't bring you anxiety or stress. It's just ten minutes. I know you can find ten minutes today and every day. Number two, this will give you enough time to see the results of the practice in your mind, your thoughts, and your energy. It really is amazing what you can do in ten minutes.

You can find this free and quick meditation on my Balboa website at www.candyholmesfoster.com. Download it and use it each day for a week. This is a great starting point that isn't too scary but is calling you to commit to yourself. How long are you willing to ignore what you really are before you grab on to your destiny and take it?

Take this one step for yourself and see where it takes you. You are the one who has to choose your path, and you are the one who needs to start the journey. Allow yourself to go within and see what your imagination has in store for you.

Research shows that only 8 percent of people achieve their dreams/goals and 92 percent just give up or fail to do it. That is a huge percentage. Are you willing to be part of the 92 percent? I hope not because I know that each and every one of us can be successful if we just believe and act on our dreams. We just need to get out of our own way. Stop believing we are just like the 92 percent and trust that we are in that 8 percent and make that percentage grow. There is no reason we cannot turn those numbers on their head and flip that coin.

Who determines who can be successful and who can't? We do. We are the ones who have to believe we can accomplish our dreams. We need to ignore those naysayers who will always try to bring us down because we are making them uncomfortable. You are the one who can; instead of getting upset when someone calls you an overachiever or wonder woman, realize that that is their problem, not yours.

When people make comments like that, it is because they feel threatened by what you are doing. They are uncomfortable with the fact that they are not going after their own dreams. I've come to realize that's a pretty good sign that you're on the right track. Just keep going. Don't let them be another reason to delay your ascension. Don't let their discomfort get in the way of your realization of your true self and your true dreams.

When I was in my first marriage, I thought being tough and working three jobs while raising my two girls and doing whatever my husband wanted, no matter the cost, was being a good wife. I thought that when he pointed out my weight problems, my lack of time and energy, and told me I couldn't manage money, he was right and I was not worthy of success of any kind.

Now I realize that I was making him uncomfortable, even back then when I didn't have any idea of who I was or what my dreams even were. I was lost in what I thought was my responsibility in our society as a mother and a wife.

Now I know I can do all those things well and still be the person I want to be. I don't have to sell my soul to be a good mom or wife. I can be who I really am and still do all that and more. In fact, now that I know I can take care of myself first and follow my dreams, I can be better at all those other things and responsibilities.

So how long will you allow your outside world to dictate whether you accomplish your dreams? Will you step up and take back the power to run your own life and reach for those dreams you've been thinking weren't possible?

I don't care how old you are. I don't care how broke you are. I don't care how many children you have or what your family thinks of you. There is a way you can take inspired action toward your dreams.

Sometimes that means keeping it quiet for a while. I know there have been several times throughout this journey where I didn't say much about the things I'd been discovering right out of the gate. Sometimes you need to get comfortable with it yourself first. Other times you may be so excited that you just have to share with someone. Choose someone you can trust to have your back and really be there for you.

It took me a long time to tell anyone that I wanted to write a book. In fact, my first book was a cookbook; it seemed a little more attainable at the time, and I am proud of that book still. I may do another one someday. Who knows? The possibilities are endless.

It took me a long time to tell anyone that my real dream was to be an Inspirational speaker and stand in front of thousands of people and be able to help them through some of the shit I've made my way through in my life. I guess I was afraid they'd think I was arrogant. But I finally did. I told my husband, and he didn't laugh at me. When I told my sister, she said, "Oh my god, I wish we lived closer to each other. Me too."

So when you're ready, share your dreams with those you know you can trust. You'll be so amazed at the responses you will get. You see, we all have big dreams if we allow ourselves to dream them. Why the heck do we always think we are not worthy of them? Why the heck do we think we are being ridiculous and outrageous?

Let's take some time to look around us and take notice of those people we follow, love, and think have it all together. Why do we think we cannot do that? Why do we think they have something we do not?

In all reality, we are ripping ourselves off with these degrading thoughts of ourselves. We are letting ourselves down by not giving ourselves enough credit to create those dreams. Why would we have those dreams if we weren't meant to bring them into the world? Our imagination is their place of origin, and those are the seeds of change.

Once we imagine them, it's our job to bring them to fruition. Doing that means taking inspired action. Water the seeds. Inspired action means acting on those impulses when they are in the moment. It doesn't matter what it is as long as it's in the direction of that dream. Sometimes one step is all you need to get that ball rolling in the right direction and at a greater and greater momentum.

Just get that ball rolling. How long are we willing to run on autopilot in the actions of what we are expected to do each day? Living in lack and sadness, in dullness, and just in a fog from day to day, doing the same things over and over again.

I know I used to go to work, come home, do more work, drink a lot, and then go to sleep or not. Now I get up in the morning, work out, meditate, go to work, come home, write or read or record or research, and then go to bed. The difference is that I start my day taking care of myself and I fit my dreams in throughout my day. I make time for the things I love like meditation and writing a book, recording meditations, surrounding myself with the things I love like books and crystals, essential oils, and cards and magic.

My life is filled with passion, and I love each day. I love my job and everything else I squeeze in around it. Yes, I'm exhausted at the end of each day, but I can truly say I'm living my life now. I don't have to worry about someone saying to me ever again, "Candy, If you don't like it, do something about it," because I already have done something about it. Thank you, GTB.

I am making my dreams come true one day at a time, and you can do the same. Do you have a moment in your past where someone said something to you that initially hurt you to the core, but later you were so glad they had the courage and love for you to tell you the truth and out you in your present situation?

If so, go there now. Bring that love for them and their courage into your heart and use that love to step into your power again. Use that person's love for you to ignite the passion within you right now to get out there and go for what you want and dream of. Take that first step toward your new life—that life you've dreamed of for so long but never thought was possible.

Use the emotion of that situation, no matter how long ago it was, to light that fire in you and step into your own personal and inner strength. Dream that dream as big as you can dream it and let it grow until you can't dream it any bigger. Dream of the details big and small and break them down into bite-sized pieces. Imagine this plan in your mind and let it play out. You can put this dream and all its details down on paper or on a vision board. Create the visual in any way that feels good for you. Just start acting on it.

14

DO, BE, AND HAVE WHAT YOU WANT!

> Life shrinks or expands in proportion with one's courage.
> —Anaïs Nin

What do you want to do, be, and have?

What do you really want? Some people, when asked this question, don't even know. All they know is, they want more. They want something other than what they have now. They truly don't know what they want, what they want to be, how they want to feel, what they want to have, and they certainly don't know how they will get there.

Of course, they don't know how they'll get there if they don't know what that is or where it is, let alone how that would feel. These are key components when you begin ascending toward your dreams. We must figure out what those dreams are.

That means we need to spend some time with ourselves. Yes, I know that to some may sound scary and ridiculous, but it's god's honest truth. You need time with you. Time to get to know yourself, love yourself, and I mean really love yourself. Then and only then will you know what you really want. Because we need to get in touch with that inner self and know that self on a visceral level. We need to accept ourselves for who we are and love ourselves for it.

I know that sounds foreign in this twenty-first century, but if you don't know who you are deep down, then how can you know what you want? So if you started the ten-minute practice mentioned in the past chapter, then you are on your way to just that. If you haven't, then what are you waiting for? You're clearly still reading so you are in, but are you fully in? If you haven't started that ten-minute practice yet, then put this book down right now and take those ten minutes to do so. I'll be happier to have you back when you're done.

OK, now that that's done, welcome back. Sometimes we need a little bit more of a shove, don't we? That's exactly why I think we all need a coach. We all need someone to give us that little extra boost we need to step up and do what needs to be done, even if it's only a ten-minute exercise that we're procrastinating on.

Believe me, I have been the queen of procrastination from time to time and sometimes for an extended period. The thing I've learned is to notice those times and use them to my advantage. When I find myself procrastinating on something, that's a sign that I need to do it right now. You may find this will serve you well too going forward.

Getting back to the matter at hand, you've started your ten-minute practice. Congratulations, now keep it going. Do it at least once per day. This is the very best way to get to know yourself. I don't care what you call it: mindfulness, meditation, concentration, time out, whatever feels good for you. It really doesn't matter what you call it. If you take that time for yourself, you will see benefit from it. Do it every day, and you'll find you crave this time. You'll want to extend your time from ten minutes to twenty and thirty, and believe it or not, you may find yourself in this place for an hour someday.

The key is to make it a regular practice for you. This is my number one form of self-care. If I miss this time in my day, something just feels off. Nothing flows like it usually does, and I don't like it.

As you get to know yourself better from the inside out, then you will start to see what it is you really want. You'll start to figure out what you want to do, what you want to be, what you want to have, *and* you'll realize that that's all OK. It is totally OK to want to do something bigger and want bigger things and nicer things in your life. It is OK.

Oftentimes that becomes a touchy subject when we're in the spiritual realm, but yes, it is OK to want things, within context. If you're here reading this, then I assume you know that things are not what it's all about, but we are allowed to want things. We are allowed to want more in our lives. Finding the line between enough and too much is what each and every one of us has to figure out.

It's another part of the journey, figuring out that perfect place and the amount of the physical stuff we invite into our lives—nothing to worry about though. This too will come with our daily practice whatever that evolves into for you, and it will evolve.

That's the point of this book: to show you the tools that I've used along my journey so far and let you know that your journey will look way different from mine. There is no right or wrong way to transcend your ascension journey. Here there are no steadfast rules. We can follow what feels good along the way.

That is also how we can start to figure out what it is we want. Try new things that pop up in your life. See what feels good and what excites you. Your life is likely already guiding you along this journey, and you may not even know it yet.

For me, Crohn's diagnosis was a pivotal point in my life, and it sent me down a path I'd never imagined. It's taken many twists and turns along the way, but I am thrilled with where it has brought me. Don't be afraid to go down that rabbit hole and see what's down there. Sometimes it won't turn up much right then and then it will come back to you later. Maybe it just didn't connect the first time around, but the second it makes total sense. Other times it just isn't for you.

I've had this happen several times. Just keep following those bread crumbs until one day you wake up and you know what you want. You are inspired and you're passionate, and you just know. You can see it in your mind.

For me, one day I could just see myself standing before the microphone on the stage in front of all the people. I could see the book. I could see the traveling to speaking engagements, and the vision gets clearer every day. This will happen to you too.

The more you get to know you, the more dreams you find come up. You can see other dreams clear as day too. You can feel the passion behind them and the reason you want them. You can feel the excitement that accompanies them, and that's what it's all about.

When you feel that passion coming in though, you must act on it. It doesn't happen all by itself, so when you can feel it, act on it. The hardest part is the first steps, so just take them and it will get easier from there.

As you take one step after the other, continue to allow yourself to feel the passion behind it. Don't allow yourself to forget that passion. Feel it all along the journey. If you feel like you've lost sight of that feeling, take a step back and assess the situation. See if it still feels good from where you are. Do you need to pivot or even step back a little?

Sometimes this is hard but it's important. Otherwise, you might all of a sudden be a long way down the road on a journey that isn't what you wanted it to be, and it feels nothing like what you had envisioned.

There will be lots of turns in the road, side steps, and side journeys along the way, but usually, it's all meant to happen. Trust the process and keep going. Never give up. Once you figure out what it is, never give up. It might take longer than you thought. It might take a different path than you thought, but never give up. Most of the time, in the end, you'll find that it turned out better than you ever imagined.

We all have the right to want what we want, be what we want, and have what we want as long as it is for the highest good and we serve in a way that lights us up. I have no doubt it can be achieved.

My very favorite prayer is "May I serve in a way that lights up my body, mind, and spirit for the highest and best good of all." I feel like that says it all. Isn't that what it's all about? We're all in this thing we call life together, and we are all here to help one another through the journey.

Do you remember that statistic from earlier? Only 8 percent of people actually do what they want to do. Looking back, why do you think that is? I think it's more because they don't know what they want than it is about actually doing it. Yes, I'm sure there are many other reasons, but I don't think it's just one reason for anyone anyway.

I think knowing what you want is another important step on this staircase that we call life. Getting to know ourselves and finding that thing that lights us up is one of those very big steps but one with so much reward if you care to take it on.

I have a meditation that will help take you through the steps of getting to know yourself better and will help you navigate these first few big steps on the staircase. You can go to my website at www.candyholmesfoster.com/bonus. This is a free download for you. I hope you enjoy it.

When you settle in for this meditation, bring a pen and paper or a journal to have handy. When you finish the meditation, go to your journal and write down what comes up for you. Then just keep writing. It doesn't matter if it makes sense. Just allow yourself to freely write whatever comes up.

You may be amazed at what ideas, thoughts, actions to take, passions you never knew you had or even thought of before. Allow it all to come out on the paper without judgment. Just write until the feed stops coming. Then and only then, go back and read it.

This practice may be the beginning of your new life's journey. I hope it inspires you into immediate action toward your goals and dreams. If nothing else, you should have an idea of something new to explore and discover, something new you want to try or experiment with. As long as it is inspired, you are on the right path.

There is no exact way that this plays out for anyone. Accept now that it will be different for you than for me. Be open to what it is and be excited to see what your journey looks like for you and you alone. I am just here to inspire you and hopefully get you headed in the right direction—the direction of your truth, of knowing you and what you want to do, be, and have in this lifetime.

Here are some inspired questions that got me moving on my journey and I hope they are helpful for you too.

What memory do you want to leave behind from this lifetime? What thing that's bigger than you do you want to be a part of while you are on this earth? How will you make a difference in this world? What talents can you share with the world? What are you passionate about? How can you share those passions? Is your passion your purpose? How are your passion and your purpose? Who can you confide in that you trust unconditionally? What are you procrastinating on right now? When will you take inspired actions on that one thing you are procrastinating on right now?

If this turns nothing up for you when you first start out, don't fret. If you're new to tapping into your higher self, this can take a minute. Here are a few exercises to get you started that might feel a little more comfortable. Don't stop trying the previous exercise though. This is a practice in listening to our higher consciousness, and it does take practice and time.

There are other ways to tap into and discover your passions. Closely connected to getting clearer on your core values, the concept of finding your true north is about discovering what motivates you. What type of impact or goal compels you? What makes you feel complete and present as if you are doing what you were made to do? Finding your true north is what some people might describe as discovering who you really are. Your true north is where your values, beliefs, and your sense of purpose meet.

Let's start by taking a look at your values. Your personal values are the things that are important to you in the way you work and live. Your values determine your personal goals and priorities. And they often act as personal indicators of whether you are a success or not.

Take some time now to consider the things that are important to you. Your values may include things like authenticity, achievement, adventure, balance, challenge, community, compassion, connection, courage, creativity, curiosity, determination, empathy, faith, fame, family, forgiveness, freedom, friendship, fun, health, honesty, inner peace, innovation, justice, kindness, knowledge, leadership, learning, love, loyalty, meaningful work, morality, nature, optimism, power, productivity, recognition, security, service, spirituality, success, trust, vitality, wealth, wisdom, and the list goes on and on.

I hope this beginning list brings some things to mind for you. What things are important to you in your life? Write it down.

Next, what do you love? This shouldn't take a lot of time. If you love it, then it will come to mind right away. Write it down.

What don't you love? This one may not be quite as quick and easy as what you love, but it shouldn't be too time-consuming. Most of us are very aware of the things we don't like. Write them down.

Next, what are you good at? Again, this shouldn't be a difficult task. We are generally aware of the things we are good at even though we tend to be more aware of the things we're not good at. Write these things down along with the others above.

Now look at all of the things you've written down and see if anything pops up for you. Allow yourself to disconnect from your normal path of thinking and focus on this list. Here's your chance to focus on logic.

In looking at this list, what comes to you as a logical option? Don't judge it. Just write it down. Don't overthink it. Just write it down.

Now go back to meditation and try it again. See what comes up now. Don't forget to do the writing activity after and see what comes up. When you're done with the meditation and you've done your free writing, take a break for a few minutes. Get up and go do something else for at least ten to fifteen minutes, longer if you wish as long as you come back to it.

Now come back to your lists, sit down, and read through them. Grab a clean sheet of paper and begin to write your vision statement. This is your personal statement of what you want to accomplish in your life. Create this vision statement around all that you've discovered during this activity.

At the end of this activity, you should have a much clearer view of what you want in life. That means what you want to do and be—what that includes, how you will get there, how it will feel when you're there, and how you are serving in a way that lights you up.

If you don't have all those details yet, keep working on it. You're getting closer all the time. No matter what, you're headed in the right direction. You're listening to your inner self and becoming more and more attuned to you. You are getting to know yourself better and better with every activity and every meditation session you participate in.

Every time you think you're getting lost as to what it is you want, take some time to think about those important things. What do you need? What makes you happy? Go back to those personal values and ask yourself, What gives me purpose? What allows me to flow? What would I rather do? Who do I want to be with? Who do I want to help? Am I where I need to be to do what I want to do? Am I willing to sacrifice to achieve my goals? What does success look like to me? What or who do I admire? Why?

This kind of questioning and self-awareness will help you understand why you feel the way you feel, what you want, and what you don't want.

Other and maybe some harder questions to ask are, What are you willing to sacrifice to achieve your goals? Are you ready to be vulnerable? Can you have courage? Are you open to change? These questions may be harder but can bring you true clarity around your goals. It's good to be ultra-aware of your boundaries and your limits.

It's also important to be super honest with yourself here. Are you *really* ready for the amount of change it might take?

15

BELIEVE

In faith, there is enough light for those who want to believe and enough shadows to blind those who don't.

—Blaise Pascal

Beliefs are our brain's way of making sense of and navigating our complex world. They are mental representations of the ways our brains expect things in our environment to behave, and how things should be related to each other—the patterns our brain expects the world to conform to.

It can seem a little confusing in the context of this chapter. True belief is a tough thing to acquire, and it is another process that takes some inner soul searching and practice. Have you noticed a pattern here? Everything we are discussing in this book takes practice. We are building one giant practice no different from a yoga or meditation practice itself. This is the practice of self-actualization.

We're talking about belief in oneself and belief in whatever we can dream is possible. Each of us having the ability to believe that our dreams are possible is a tall order for most. I know I spent many years saying that I believed I could accomplish my goals, create my dreams, and manifest my wildest dreams. I was lying to myself. I'm grateful that I've walked along this path long enough and can honestly say that I do believe I can accomplish my dreams, create my destiny, and be the cocreator of my world.

Yes, it has taken constant practice and, might I say, a lot of "fake it until you make it" kind of stuff too. I mean, if you don't believe fully in yourself but you want to believe in yourself, then that's the only way to get there, right?

There has been many a ride to work and back listening to Louise Hay's book *I Can Do It*[9] and reciting all the affirmations over and over again. I may not have believed them at the time, but I kept doing it until I did. Now when I say, "Abundance flows effortlessly into all areas of my life," I am 100 percent telling the truth.

It's almost like building a wall of strength with all your practices that create the belief in yourself. So many of us go through life with injured selves deep within. There is work to be done to heal those wounds, and for most of us, it's a practice of trial and error.

I've known for years that I had deep issues surrounding money and my own worth. I've used many practices to heal those wounds that stretch back through my lineage. I don't feel they are fully healed yet, but I honestly can say I am making headway. I am making progress and becoming a more functional and better-evolved person for it.

I tell you this because I think it's important to know that we're all going through something, battling something, or working on something that may seem unending and that thing that weighs us down and keeps us trapped in that muck. I am no different from you or your neighbor. We are all in this thing together, and I am here to share with you my experience in the hopes that it can help you in any small way.

Our belief systems begin in our childhood and evolve through the things we are taught are right or wrong. Sometimes as we grow older and step out into the world, we can be disheartened when we find that those things we were taught may not be quite as rock solid as we once thought.

This happens to many in many ways. Someone you looked up to may fall from your grace with just one action that is shocking. Sometimes the whole basis of a belief system rears its ugly head and you suddenly see it for what it really is. Still other times, a person or thing that you've idolized for your lifetime shows their true light, and your heart is broken. This is when we don't know what to believe. This is when we feel stuck and lost.

Yet this is also when you can start from scratch. Start from the bottom to explore and investigate and find out what *you* believe. It can happen. That is how I evolved into my belief system today, by starting at the bottom.

Our belief system around a higher power can be a very tender subject. I know that is an area where I was disheartened as a young adult and ignored it because I didn't know what to believe anymore.

I did not raise my children teaching them any specific rules of God or religion because I felt like I had no right to do so when I didn't know what I really believed myself. Just because I was raised in a certain religion didn't mean I should raise my children the same.

I did feel guilty about that for some time as my girls got older. But later they thanked me for not pushing them along any one path. They as well as I have been able to find what I think is the perfect view of our higher power.

I believe that we all worship the same god. That god just looks different to each and every one of us. My studies of religious history have helped me come to this understanding. There is a deep connection between most of the religions of the world where things spill over from one to the other and most of the principles are the same. Be a good person. Isn't that what it's all about? Be a decent human being while you're here on this earth, share your light, and make this stay a meaningful one.

That means doing something you're proud of and sharing it with the world. This is where bringing our god beliefs into our self-beliefs is a huge tool in our ascension. Learning how to believe in yourself, your worth, your abilities, and all the possibilities will take you a long way on this journey of manifesting the life you desire. Let's learn how to believe.

As I mentioned, affirmations were a major tool on the journey to believing in myself. Believing in my worthiness and believing in my ability to create this life and do the things that back then felt so big and out of my reach.

Why do we automatically feel that those things we dream of are not attainable? Well, what does your track record look like? Some people set goals, but month after month, make no progress, lie to themselves, and don't seem to care. But if you build a habit of breaking your own promises, you'll gradually stop believing in yourself, lose confidence, and lose hope, which makes it even harder to achieve your goals.

This is where I have found affirmations that got me started on the right path. Then I started to focus on only making promises to myself that I could and would keep. Failing to keep promises to yourself hurts your self-belief. Studies show that keeping promises holds a lot of emotional value—and when we break those agreements, there's a decline in trust.

Each time we keep a promise to ourselves, we show ourselves that we are trustworthy, we uphold our word, and we can confidently rely on ourselves to follow through on our commitments.

So why is it we're more likely to break a promise to ourselves than we are to someone else? Well, most likely no one else will know but you and most of us care what others think of us. So we're more likely to sacrifice ourselves to the cause. We're also creatures of immediate satisfaction, and when we don't see the results we want quickly enough for our liking, we tend not to follow through.

This is where a lack of focus can bring us down in a quick hurry. Staying focused on our goals and dreams takes work. Life keeps happening whether we have goals or not. That means even though our world stays busy and stressful at times, we need to find a way to stay focused and make time to keep moving forward with those inspired actions and those promises that we make to ourselves.

As I write these words, I realize that I have let this happen throughout the writing of this book. I made a pledge to myself to write 2,000 words a day five days a week in order to keep moving forward in manifesting my dream of writing this book. I had a goal of having the rough draft done by 8/8 (the lion's gate portal's peak energy day). Today is 7/21, and I am behind on my quota because I've let life get in the way over the past few weeks.

Now I need to up the ante from my original goal and need to get 2,300 words per day. This is only because I had a day all to myself and did 7,000 yesterday. The point is now I must pay the price and work even harder not to break my own promise to myself, which would be a detrimental move in my own self-realization.

Another thing about focus is that many of us have too many goals. We try to achieve a million different things at once, yet every goal has an opportunity cost; doing one thing usually takes time and energy away from another.

I talked earlier about the book *Eat That Frog*. That book has been helpful for me in this process, because it has helped me focus on my three main goals for the day and anything above and beyond that is just gravy. Top three every day is my focus though.

There is a thing called Parkinson's law of triviality, which is when we spend more time on insignificant tasks and less time on the things that are more impactful on our end goals. I remember when I was in health coach school and I was working on my business, my website, and my program itself, they told us, "It will never be perfect, so just do it." There is some real truth to this action. We often nitpick and primp and polish the little details to death and never get our dreams off the ground when we're playing this game.

Focus on what really gets the things done and creates progress. Spend your time on the 20 percent of things that will create 80 percent of your results. That way, you get the biggest impact from your effort and move forward faster.

This is closely related to perfectionism. We will never have it perfect, so there is a point when we need to move forward versus revamping certain details over and repeatedly.

Accountability is a huge hurdle for many people. It's hard to stay accountable to yourself, just like it's easier to break a promise to yourself. Who will know other than you? Exactly—you will know, so keep yourself accountable; it will be worth it in the end. There are many ways to do this. Confide in someone who will help you in this area. My husband keeps me accountable to myself because I know that he knows this is my dream and if he sees me not doing what I need to do, he'll be on me like flies on rice.

I do love him for it though. I can always count on him to be there when I need a little shove, a nudge, or even a kick in the backside. He knows what my dreams are, and he also knows me better than anyone else in this world. He knows my strengths and my weaknesses, and he helps me be stronger in those weaker areas.

If you don't have someone in your life like that, you could hire a coach. I'm a firm believer that we all need a coach in some area of our lives. Maybe this is your area. This is a true investment in yourself. There are also apps out there to keep you accountable for your goals; there are journals and planners of every type out there as well. Just be careful not to fall into that Parkinson's law pitfall when it comes to journaling, planning, and replanning. Find what works for you and keeps you moving forward.

Another thing that holds us back is often our environment. Is your environment conducive to what you are trying to accomplish? It's not productive for me to sit down to write in the evening after dinner when I'm clearly tired and worn down and while my husband is watching WWE. I'm already tired and clearly not full of inspiration, and even though I couldn't care less about wrestling, I will be distracted.

I know for a fact I'm much better off going at it in the morning before I go to work or even while dinner is cooking before John gets home when it's nice and quiet and there are no distractions.

Surrounding yourself with the environment you need to be focused on and that nurtures your inspiration and concentration is key. I also know that my best time to work out is first thing in the morning. I know and have proven this repeatedly throughout the years. The longer I wait to do my workout, the less likely it is to happen. Therefore, I get up in the morning, hydrate, and go to work out—period. This leaves no time for overthinking, and excuses. I just do it. That is the environment I've created, and I refuse to break that pattern because I do have a history of not being consistent in this area.

Look at your goals now. Does your environment assist you in accomplishing these goals? What might need to change? This can be a number of things, including your physical environment, the time you allow for working toward your goal, financial allowances, and planning—or is it strategic planning? Only you know what this looks like. Assess the situation and make the changes that need to be made for your own success. You're worth it.

Fear is the other biggie when it comes to not attaining your goals. There is actually a thing called fear of success as well as that fear of failure. Achieving your goals could create difficult outcomes or emotions—jealous friends, the realization you never wanted it, guilt, etc.—so some people inadvertently sabotage their own progress.

Second, some attach their self-worth to their goals. That means if they give their best effort and fail, it will devastate them and reflect on their character. As a result, they might make a half-hearted effort, so any resulting failure is less damaging to their ego—or they'll work on trivial things (i.e., bike shedding) to avoid finishing and facing possible rejection.

Fear is a huge hurdle no matter which end of the spectrum you reside at. Fear can consume us and keep us from moving forward at all. Facing our fears takes commitment and focus—and laser focus, at that. It takes leaving no room for excuses and being very present with all your thoughts and actions.

Give yourself some time today while in your ten-minute meditation to assess where fear is showing up in your life. This time is the best time to do this as in your meditative state, you're more able to see things objectively and without judgment. Ask yourself, How am I living in fear? Where is fear showing up in my life and how is it holding me back?

Now that we have all these hurdles out in the open, where do we begin? Right at the beginning. Let's take our activities from the past chapters and pull all that information together.

We're not going to spend a ton of time on this, but this is some foundational work that needs to be done to avoid all the things we have just discussed. Take that information and read it through again. Where do you see yourself inadvertently sabotaging your efforts? Bring awareness to your habits, tendencies, and those things you know about yourself that will not serve you well going forward.

Let's bring forward our strengths and weaknesses and plan to utilize those strengths to their fullest and create a plan to combat those weaknesses. As we become more aware of our own actions and tendencies, we can create an environment where true belief in ourselves monopolizes our thinking and every activity in the making of our dreams.

This is not something that just happens; it is something we create for ourselves. Once we achieve the belief in ourselves and the possibilities we can create, we can achieve any goals we put our minds to.

Once we believe in ourselves and we believe that anything we can dream is possible, then we can manifest anything our hearts desire that is in alignment with our true self and the highest good of all; and we're willing to do the work. That means being aware and present and knowing that this is truly *your* dream, not the dreams of someone else: parents, partners, friends. This must be yours and yours alone. You must own it and love it and feel it in your heart.

This belief really comes into play when we're working on our manifestations, whether physically doing the work or doing our power-of-attraction work practices. As you can see, we need both. It doesn't work with belief and no action. It also doesn't work with action and no belief. If you don't believe you can get there, then you surely will not. It's as plain and simple as that. That is why we need to start here and build up our belief in ourselves and our ability as well as our worthiness.

If you are trying to manifest that you'll win a million dollars, but you never buy a ticket, then you certainly are not going to win. In the same right, if you are trying to manifest that same million-dollar winning ticket and you buy that ticket but really don't believe you'll win, then the same holds true. It won't happen.

Remembering what we think about what we bring about, even if no one else knows what we're thinking—this is the pinnacle of the law of attraction. You must believe it, you must feel it, and you must imagine it. See it in your mind.

In Wayne Dyer's book *Excuses Begone*,[10] he talks about there being nothing in our lives that we cannot change. He goes on to talk about everything being about choices, and when we say we have no choices, we are just making excuses. Those are pretty strong statements, but if you think about that statement for a while, you will find that he is 100 percent correct. There are always choices in every situation. Sometimes we don't like the ones we are presented with, but they are choices nonetheless.

Making the decision to hold yourself accountable for everything that goes on in your life is practice. This will create a deeper belief in oneself; it has for me. Once I stopped making excuses for the things in my life and accepted that I have created this life and I am the only one with the power to change it, my outlook on the whole picture changed.

The day I decided that the basket of candy in the back room had no control over me and I did have control over me was the day I stopped making excuses for my weight. The day I stopped saying I was going to write a book and started writing a book was the day I started to believe that I could write the book. The day two weeks later when the Balboa Press called, I believed it a little more. The day my husband said, "Yes, let's do this self-publishing package with Balboa Press," I believed a lot more. As I near the end of my rough draft and am looking at a rough mockup of the cover, I believe even more.

This is how we build on the power of our belief, literally building it one stone at a time—one successful thought, one successful manifestation, one strategic move at a time that takes you closer and closer to the actualization of your goals.

So keep taking those steps, getting rid of those excuses, visualizing your goals, and being present with your emotions. Keep moving forward and never give up. Allow your belief system to back up your belief in yourself. Believe you are worthy of all you can imagine. Why else would you be able to imagine it? This is what you're meant for. Each and every one of us is meant to actualize our dreams. In the brutally unforgettable words of Wayne Dyer, *excuses begone!*

That is not to say we need to go it alone. Something else that can help us believe in ourselves a little more is incorporating that higher power that we discussed earlier. Putting our faith in that can allow us to trust and believe on a different level, letting go of the notion that it is all up to us and only we can get it done.

So even though we have the ability to make choices, dismiss excuses, and walk the walk to make those changes in our lives, we are certainly never alone. We always have the ability to leave it in God's hands. That can increase our level of belief immensely.

I'd love to have you take some time now to assess your goals and your level of belief in attaining those goals. Which ones need some work and which ones are you feeling confident in? Are there some that you feel you need to let go now, that just don't feel right anymore? That can also be a reality.

Be present with what comes up and be honest with yourself. This is an opportunity to better focus your energy on what is important to you and let go of the things that no longer are serving you on this journey.

Where can you upgrade your environment to optimize your progress and where are you willing to sacrifice somewhere else to accommodate the time you need to attain your goals?

Do you have too many goals you're trying to attain right now? Do you need to let some go or put them on hold for a short time? I certainly have a couple of goals I've been working on together, and I have found it hard to fit them both in. The writing of this book and attaining my sports nutrition certification are fighting for time, and I often have to take a moment to prioritize.

I continue to work on attaining my certification, but this book takes precedence over all else, so for this week, in order to hit my current goal, the class has to go on hold. It will be there next week when I have more time to devote to it. For right now, I must focus solely on getting my rough draft done.

Allow yourself to think outside the box and really be honest with yourself. Sometimes it comes down to a simple question. Which one is more important to you overall? Even though you may be passionate about both projects (or more), sometimes a decision needs to be made in order to make progress at all and not get bogged down by all that needs to be done and burn us out.

Sometimes we just spend our time spinning our wheels in the muck of too many projects instead of putting all our focus and efforts into one. At the same time, we can leave the rest in the universe's capable hands and it will likely all work out in the end.

I find the more I let go and trust that all will be fine, the more it is. The words "Trust unconditionally" rate right up there with "Believe" when it comes to difficulty in getting there, but when you do, there's no turning around. You will for life once you figure it out.

If we continue to trust unconditionally and believe unconditionally, we're going to make it a place. We're going to make it to all the places we ever dreamed of and most likely even more. I love to add the phrase "or better" to all my prayers just because I know that I haven't even begun to imagine all that I am capable of, but my higher power certainly does know what that is.

Our higher power knows more than we can imagine in our entire lifetimes. If we just trust and believe that we've been given the ability to accomplish whatever we can imagine, then we can meet any goal we could possibly set for ourselves.

16

WE MUST TAKE INSPIRED ACTION

Don't let what you cannot do interfere with what you can do.
—John Wooden

The one thing I think so many people miss when it comes to achieving their dreams and manifesting their desires is the importance of action. Let's be realistic—most of the time, things don't happen purely because we want them to.

Yes, there is that aspect of manifestation where we must want it and feel it to create it, but almost always there is some kind of action that needs to take place on our part to get things rolling. Even if it's winning the lottery, you still must buy the ticket in order to win.

After I received my certification in mindfulness meditation years ago, I had to take those first steps to put myself out there. I had to step out of my comfort zone and tell the world I was teaching meditation classes, and let me tell you, in a small town in northern New Hampshire, that was a big step. I thought everyone might think I'd lost my mind, but I knew I needed to share this with the world. I had to share what this could do for everyone. So I had to act.

The same thing held true when John and I moved to the southern part of the state at the beginning of 2020. I had to let people know that I was here and my business was here to help people, even in the middle of a pandemic. How the heck do I do that? Well, I did that in the most uncomfortable way possible. I started cold-calling people in our new town.

Yes, that would be the first thing I would do when I stepped into my office in the morning. I would call five more people. Full disclosure here, I hated every single one of them until I started to connect with some people who wanted to talk to me. I started to meet some neat people, and I think sometimes it even made their day because we couldn't see anyone at that time. It felt good to connect with like-minded people in this new world of mine.

My business never took off again once we moved here, but I know there were other lessons and progress made for me at that time. If nothing else, I stepped out of my comfort zone and gave that business everything I had. And by taking those steps outside that comfy circle, I made that comfort zone bigger.

Fast-forward to now and I'm coaching and helping more people than I could have ever reached with my little business in my little town. That means the action I took when my business just wasn't taking hold was to apply for a job even though I really didn't want to give up on that dream. Thank you, universe.

Now I know that when I had my own business, I had to be the accountant, the marketing girl, the creator, the advertiser, the tech guy, the buyer, and eventually the coach. I was spending more time on all the other parts of my business than I was helping people to feel better. Now I don't have any of those headaches on my plate, and I can focus on what I do best: help people.

That also gives me the time and energy before and after work to create more inspired action. I have the energy to create new meditations and record, edit, and upload them. I have the energy and inspiration to write a book and make sure I write every day. When I do, I keep that channel open and active, and I keep those creative juices flowing. It also creates good habits, consistency, and progress.

There were other ways that I created inspired action during those COVID shutdown days. I also started doing a live Facebook meditation every morning at 7:00 a.m. I started with a free thirty-day challenge and then transitioned into a monthly membership group. I certainly wasn't making a ton of money doing it, but I was doing what I loved and it felt good to help people feel better at a time when we all felt truly isolated and alone.

That action helped me too. I was also home alone and isolated. I'm so glad that task brought me together with even a select few people during that time. Even though it was all online, I feel truly connected to those ladies still today. When we take action, we do it for a particular result. Anytime you intentionally act, it is all because of the desired outcome. Execute your actions to support your dreams and goals, and you never know what might come out of it.

Failure to act can stem from many areas, the main one being the failures of the past. If we look at our failures as a lesson learned though, we may be willing to learn even more. Stretching us beyond what we can see builds trust within ourselves and grabs hold of the present.

In the situations above especially, I have found that when I take specific actions, it helps me shift and pivot. If COVID did nothing else, it did force all of us to do this in one way or another. Then oftentimes when we pivot or change our direction, it ignites new motivation. It excites us or re-excites us.

Continued action can also create habits of action, which in turn create more action. When I was making those phone calls, I never started looking forward to them, but it did become a habit. It was just what I did when I got in the office every single day. No questions asked and consistent actions equal consistent progress.

Our actions create results as a chain reaction. Sometimes those results are not what we want or expect, but they are results just the same. A chain reaction, though even a disappointing result, moves you on to the next step in the process. There's no point beating a dead horse, right? Moving on—that in turn silences our inner criticism—that voice inside us that we're not doing enough, the right thing, or anything at all. Action gets things done way faster than sitting around, waiting for things to happen. There is an equation to this. Did you know that? Yes, the success equation to life is knowledge plus action equals success. So let's gain knowledge, take action, and claim success.

Ready yourself to make a commitment that removes the missing link and promotes success by acting. Here is where you will celebrate success often. The results and outcomes may not always be as expected, but a little suspense never hurts any journey.

Allow your heart to compound the experiences, including your commitment to taking that action and the results of what's to come. Claim your ultimate success when action meets you every day.

Your journey is a path of many colors. Take a chance by choosing the action that serves your purpose. Cheers to you for acting and creating your own success this new season! The best is yet to come. Be present. Be incredible. Be you!

The reality is we'll never know it all. No matter where we start, we'll always have something to learn. But we also have to be aware that seeking knowledge is holding us back. Sometimes, this is our fear rearing its ugly head again, and other times, it's that unworthiness showing up again.

That being said, I have spent much of my life collecting knowledge. You might say I am the queen of certifications. First of all, I do love to learn, but for many years, I felt like I was never ready to put myself out there. I never knew enough about this or that. Once upon a time, I felt like I needed a certification in everything under the sun.

Now I know different things. I still am always learning but more so for my own enjoyment. I often tell people, "I just geek out over this stuff," and I honestly do. I can't get enough of all the information out there on our emotional, spiritual, and physical well-being. I am always trying to put all the pieces of the puzzle together just a little better.

Today though, when I have a new idea, I dive right in and take real action. I often must pause and learn something along the way and probably more than once, but I'm constantly in action toward my goals and I find that it creates a real sense of flow in all my projects. I think it helps me keep moving forward better than before because before, I wasn't really getting started. I was always preparing.

Now I know why they call it inspired action. The point is to act when you're inspired and in the moment. Make it happen and get it started when you are excited about it and all those great ideas are in your head. It works so much better than trying to remember what that meditation was that I came up with the other day. Why can't I remember how excited I was when that came to me? It's never the same three days later. It's definitely not the same when you never get back to it and the idea is gone like the wind.

I have gotten so I always keep a notebook with me so I can scribble down some notes when I have those great ideas and then when I have a minute, as soon as I can, I can go get the whole idea down on paper. Some people do this; others use their notes app on their phone or even on their computer. Whatever works for you, this is another form of that inspired action taking place when you can't fully dive into that moment.

Sometimes dividing your project up into sections can help keep your action steps moving along. When writing a book, I start with the table of contents and then break it down from there. It's not so overwhelming when you're looking at it one chapter at a time, 2,000 words per day, or even a page a day. The same holds true when taking a class. Whatever your project looks like and however you break it out, just find a way to plot your strategy.

What do your dreams and goals look like? Can you write a table of contents or plan? It's almost like building a business plan. You start with the big picture and break it down into sections. From there, decide what tasks need to be done for each section and what kind of time and resources you'll need to get them each done.

Once you get to this point, you can start at the first section. Start at the beginning and keep knocking off one task at a time. Set yourself a timeline or a deadline. This can give you inspiration and intention, keeping an eye on the prize. This type of tactic makes everything so much less overwhelming and much more attainable.

When I take a class, the table of contents is already done for me. I set my deadline and then figure out what I must get done to attain that deadline. Or sometimes it's the other way around. Maybe I will assess the chapters and length, how many there are, and how much time I have to devote to this project and the timeline options and go from there.

There are so many ways to get your action plan in place and keep you inspired along the way. Often though, at this stage of any project, this is not your focus. In fact, the idea is quite the opposite. Usually when you are in the spontaneous mode and just getting the ideas out of your head and on paper, that is your only goal. So do that.

Fussing about the details and perfection at this point will only hinder your progress, get you stuck in your head, consume a lot of time, and drain your energy. Keep it simple at this point and get the basics down. You can go back and dress it up and get everything perfected later. You don't want to lose that momentum.

Once you get it into its rough form, then you can delve into the next step of changing, primping, and perfecting the product at hand. This will take more attention to detail, and you might like this process better or worse than the last phase, depending on your personality, your project, or your dream itself.

Nonetheless, it's part of the process and another phase and form of action needed to bring your dreams to fruition. No matter what your dreams are, this kind of process can be super helpful in bringing the whole thing down to manageable terms.

So what is your big dream? How can you take inspired action on that dream now? Is it sitting down at this moment and making this plan and breaking it down into manageable steps? I know this may feel like a form of procrastination, but it is usually a necessary part of the process if you are serious about achieving those big dreams that have always felt just too big for you. This is a way to break it down into bite-sized pieces and really see how it can be manageable and truly doable. The key is to keep moving forward in the process and stay in motion. This in turn starts to make it feel like you can attain your dream.

I would advise you to take the time now to start this. Do your big vision and then start the breakdown process into sections and then those sections into the steps needed to get there. Set yourself a timeline. When do you want each step to be completed and set a final goal for your project or manifestation?

Then start! Just start at the beginning and take that first step. Commit to the time and work you need to do each day, and before you know it, you'll have that dream in sight or even fully accomplished.

I've used this tactic repeatedly in my life, and it has served me well. I used this when planning my wedding to John when I was working on my bachelor's degree in business. I continued to use this in health coach school, starting my business, moving into our new home, and getting my personal trainer certification, and I'm using it now to complete this book. As you can see, it's a pretty flexible plan of action and helps keep you motivated and on task.

Of course, none of us are perfect, and sometimes we'll get off track and life will get in our way. Sometimes a plan needs to be adjusted, and things pop up that we did not expect or plan for—no worries. When we have a plan, at least we know where we stand, and we can adjust accordingly.

The point is to keep the ball rolling and keep moving on your journey to fulfilling your dreams. There will always be roadblocks. That's part of life; part of our challenges in life is to overcome them and keep pushing forward.

Inspired action also keeps us feeling good about our project and our progress. As we keep moving forward, we feel like our dreams really are attainable and we really can achieve anything we put our minds to. As we move through our timeline, we also create a new trust in ourselves—the trust that we will do what we say we will do.

Our dreams are why we were put here on this planet. If not, what would be the purpose? There would be none. Why would God create a whole planet of humans and animals if there was no purpose to accomplish anything of real satisfaction and joy? We all have our own purpose in this life, and achieving those and walking that path is important to making this life a success.

Success is defined as the accomplishment of an aim or purpose. Though in some people's minds success is all about money and things, I believe that success is just as it's defined and doesn't have to have anything to do with money, things, or fame.

I believe that is one of the keys to creating true success when you find that thing that brings you so much joy—that you will do it even without money or fame to accompany it. I have observed that when you do it just because you love it and you keep doing it just because you love it, then it turns into a path to abundance naturally.

Living our passion and putting our sincere energy into that which we truly love emanates out to the rest of the world, and they can feel that energy in what we do. That is what attracts others to us. Sincerity and passion come through in our work, no matter what that work is.

Sometimes you'll also be amazed at the help that arrives the moment you start taking that inspired action. When you immerse yourself in that which you truly love, the synchronicities will follow.

I'd worked on this book on and off for a couple of years now but never really got serious about it until a few months ago. Then I told myself, "This book isn't going to write itself." That day, I decided to write every day. And I did.

Within a week, I received the call from Balboa Press, and my husband approved of moving forward with the project. He was there to support me in my dream. That in itself was even more motivating because now I know he believes in me, so I'm certainly not going to let him down when he has invested in my success.

The timing was crazy, and I knew that it had all been manifested and it keeps moving forward in that same manner today. Every morning when I do my meditation and prayers, I pray for flow in writing, that the inspiration keeps coming to me. I know that I am guided by the inspiration and flow of words that get down on the paper. There are so many times I reread these pages. I'm amazed at what is here. I don't always remember writing them down. But it's good and I feel good about being a channel for this information.

I am blessed with my guides and higher self, who assist me along the way. But it still takes me sitting my butt down and doing the work. I have to put the words down that I receive, and if I don't, then it is just wasted insight and is all just lost to inspiration.

That is another thing that keeps me on task. I know that I am being guided to put this information out there for you. It is my duty to share the information with anyone who wants and needs it, whether through my books, my coaching, or my meditations. That is what I was put here for.

If I were to ignore the insight that I receive, then I would be disrespecting God, my guides, and my higher self for all that they have provided for me on this journey. Know that your passions and dreams are guided as well by that thing bigger than you. This is just one more reason to follow those dreams and keep acting. They are here to assist and will guide you along the way. It is amazing how many times I'm lost for words and feel stuck, but when I settle in and invite my higher self to assist me with the words, they suddenly appear and easily flow onto the pages.

That is what it takes to act. Find your space and go there when it's time to work on your dreams. When you need assistance and run into roadblocks, ask for help. Your higher power is always there to assist you in moving forward with ease.

I have this conversation with clients all the time when it comes to weight loss. Weight loss is not all about food. There's a lot more that goes into it. A lot of it is stuff that's stuck in our heads from past experiences, family history, and even past lives. But it takes action to work through that stuff. It takes action to face those demons and feel those pains so that you can let them go and move forward on your wellness journey.

We'll talk more about this in the emotional and physical areas of this book, but suffice it to say that action comes in many forms. Sometimes it is writing or making a plan. Other times it is letting yourself feel the feelings that have been beat down for years or even generations. Those things create blocks in our path, and we need to dig in to overcome them.

Take a moment now to think about the things that have blocked your progress so far. What are some things that you think will be hard to overcome in accomplishing your dream? Being aware of these things is important and is very helpful in the planning process. Then we can work on ways to overcome them. Planning and strategy are key, but if you aren't aware of an issue or you just don't want to see it, then you will not overcome it.

My morning meditation brings me so much awareness in all areas of my life. It allows me to stop the constant chatter, allows information and intuition to flow, and makes room for solutions to come with ease_as I need them.

This allows me to act accordingly and keep moving forward. Find your perfect time of day when you are the most productive. As for me, I'm a morning person and I tend to get more done for my personal goals and wellness before I go to work than I probably get accomplished in the rest of the day altogether.

I am most energized in the morning, so I focus on the things that are most important to me. I get my physical work done by getting my workout and my walk-in right off the bat. Then I meditate, and then if I have time, I will sit down and write for an hour. I will also write during my lunch break and sometimes when I get home from work, but the mornings are the best time for me and I know once I leave the house, at least I've done the most important things before I even start my day. It's already a successful day no matter what. It also starts my day in a higher vibration, which I crave.

Inspired action first thing in the morning is the best way for me. Everyone is different though, so assess your day and see when your most energized time of the day is. Some people get their second wind when they get home from work. Others do well late at night. It doesn't matter as long as it works for you and you utilize that time. Then you are using the gifts you've been given.

17

FIGURING OUT THE PHYSICAL

> Our bodies are our gardens—our wills are our gardeners.
> —William Shakespeare

So far, we've been focused on the very closely connected emotional and spiritual pillars of wellness. Our third pillar of physical wellness really brings it all together. I have always been passionate about wellness throughout my adult life. In my twenties, I lifted weights and was in the gym many days per week and was out for a run by five, though when I think back now, I think it was probably for all the wrong reasons. I was always trying to live up to the expectations of others, and at that age, I wanted to please everyone. So when someone told me that I didn't work hard enough and I was fat and lazy, I took that to heart.

Looking back, I should have gotten mad and told them to take a hike, but instead, I got mad and got to work. My tendency is to prove people wrong, which doesn't always work out in my favor. Sometimes it does, though.

I was always looking for compliments, I assume now, because I wasn't receiving them at home. I did feel better when I worked out regularly, and I felt better about myself as well. Intensity was my thing, but consistency could have been used for some work. This is a tendency that I still struggle with today: consistency.

I no longer live in that kind of environment, but consistency has taken it hard since I have moved on. Though it wasn't healthy, it kept me more accountable. So in recent years, I've made it a point to hold myself accountable and be much more consistent in my training.

That is one of the things that make me so proud of my oldest daughter. She also lifts weights and is a true role model for young women everywhere. She is beyond consistent with her workouts and her meal planning but has also found a balance in life as well. She is full of life and vitality, and she inspires me every day to stay on my program and keep moving forward.

This is part of the reason I decided to become a personal trainer. If there's one thing I realized a few years ago when following my passions and my purpose, usually it involves the thing you've had the most trouble with. I became a health coach because of my Crohn's disease. I am a good weight loss coach because I've struggled so much with my weight. So why wouldn't I be a good fitness coach? I've certainly struggled there too, and it will also keep me more accountable.

Our physical health affects every area of our lives, and the purpose for including it in this book is to bring a true balance of holistic wellness to our lives. I know when I am physically active, I feel much better emotionally and spiritually as well. The same holds true for the other two pillars respectively.

Just like anything else, this will look different for all of us, depending on where we are in our physical health journey. Some may be at the beginning and others may be longtime fitness advocates, whereas some, like me, may be at the beginning *again*.

My goal now is to stay consistent and improve my physical wellness gradually over time. I have always been one of those all-or-nothing people, and I'm constantly going all in on something I'm passionate about but then burning myself out or even hurting myself so that I can't continue. Then we're off again. That is my goal, to help you find your consistency.

I've always said I was going to live to be one hundred. My husband doesn't understand why I would want to do that. Well, if I was healthy and felt good, why wouldn't I? That in itself is the difference.

I have come to the realization recently though that I have not been on track to obtain that, at least not like I want it to be. If I'm going to live to be one hundred, then I want to feel good doing so. I just finished reading *Outlive: The Science and Art of Longevity*, by Peter Attia MD,[11] and he brings up several good points about prevention and preparation for living well in our later years. It has been just one more thing to light the fire of consistency under my butt.

My main goal here is to live as long as I can as well as I can. I've watched too many relatives who sat down in their recliner the day they retired and got sicker and sicker from there forward. I want to create a lifestyle now that I'm excited to submerge myself into on that day, a lifestyle I'm excited to dive into the day I retire.

Dr. Peter Attia says if we want to pick up our twenty-five-pound grandchild at seventy-five or eighty or even beyond, then we need to be able to lift forty-five pounds over our head now. That is an eye-opener now, isn't it? Even though I feel like I'm doing pretty good at getting my workouts each week and my walk on most days, I think I still need a little work.

Thankfully, this isn't a sprint, and whatever improvements we can make create a better tomorrow. If there is one thing I've learned over the years, it's to take things a little slower and steadier, and I usually make much better progress.

So what's your vision of your physical health as you age? Some people don't give this much thought, but we really need to. Making some gradual changes now will make all the difference in the world when we actually arrive at this much sought-after period of our lives. Let's do it with some vigor.

Take a moment now to assess your current fitness picture. Do you feel you are in pretty good shape, or does it need some work? What is your vision of your physical fitness at or after retirement or just as you age? Another thing many of us never take the time to visualize. I know I never did. Even though I always said I was going to live to be one hundred, I'd never really visualized what that looked like in my body.

Yes, I saw myself traveling and feeling good, but I didn't think about what it would take to get me there and what that meant physically right now. I've gone about most of my life living in a proactive state, but here I think I might have missed the mark until now.

I am a firm believer that prevention is key, especially when it comes to disease. "Food is medicine" is something that has often come out of my mouth. Yet I never took that train of thought when it came to fitness and my overall longevity.

Yes, we all know that regular cardio will help strengthen our heart, and weight-bearing exercise can strengthen our bones, but do we really picture this in our lives? I have not. I hadn't until then anyway. I'm assuming, like most of us, you're more focused on the here and now, right?

Unfortunately, a lot of the time the now wins out, and the later rewards of exercise and fitness don't always overpower crashing on the couch at the end of the day. This is how it all begins. So let's head that off at the past by creating a vision of what we want in this arena is important as well. Once we create that vision, we know what to aim for, and we can start to create the steps we need to get there. As you can see, this is not that different from the other areas of our life.

When our physical body is functioning properly, we sleep better, we move better, we think better, we feel better, and we manifest better. It rounds off the perfect package—this amazing package that was given to each of us and in faith that we would take good care of it all. The saying "My body is a temple" is no joke physically, emotionally, or spiritually.

We have been given these amazing gifts. Let's make the best out of each of them and all of them as a whole. By the time we're done here, we will be able to pick out some of the habits we've been making throughout our lives and make some sense of why we do them. Then we can make a plan of how to remove the ones that do not serve us anymore or ever have.

This morning, I had a session with a client who is a minister. She confessed to me that she had fallen off her program and she didn't even understand why. She had been at an art show this weekend. Something she was very passionate about was her art. On her way home drenched in rain and soaked to the bone, she stopped and got herself a coffee and a donut.

She exclaimed, "I don't even like donuts! I don't understand why I even did that. And I knew it the whole time I was eating it." Intuition came through to me that she was using the food to get grounded. This is something that many of us do when we spend a lot of time in the spiritual world. Our heads are in the clouds so much that we intuitively have to find a way to get grounded and stay in the physical world we are actually in. This is just one example of the ways that we can sabotage our own efforts without even realizing it sometimes.

Once we are able to identify those things, then hopefully we recognize them the next time around and choose differently. We can choose to get out in nature, go for a walk, a run, or a hike. Just doing something physical will distract and ground us.

She did tell me that the next morning, she went out and spent the day in her garden and left all her other agenda behind. Next time, hopefully, she'll recognize the feeling and do the gardening first.

This is her great way to get some exercise. I'm a gardener as well, and you can get some great exercise working in the garden. You don't have to go to the gym or run countless miles to get fit and healthy. Almost always, there is a way to get your exercise in by doing something you love, and I truly recommend it.

Though I do love my gym workouts, I also love taking the dog for a walk or a run. I'm a true fan of getting the work around home done with my husband. This weekend, we spent much of the weekend painting the house. That may not seem like much, but it is climbing up and down ladders and it definitely works muscles you may not work on an ordinary basis.

One of the things that has been proven to affect our health in progressive countries is that we don't do our own work anymore. The more money we make, the less physical work we tend to do, not necessarily out of laziness, but more so out of time restraints. John and I talk about that a lot. There have been many times that I thought about getting a housekeeper or hiring someone to mow the lawn, but usually, we come back to getting it done ourselves. The more we can continue to do ourselves, the more we will continue to progress in our health as well.

Plus, these are also things that can help keep us grounded. There's nothing more grounding and humbling than cleaning a toilet or a shower or doing the dishes (all my least favorite chores). Though these may seem like minute little tasks, they are still moving and take effort, and that is always better than settling into the recliner for the next ten years, wondering why you are getting sicker and sicker.

Humbling is the task that we hate, right? Keeping us grounded and keeping us real, physical work is a great equalizer. It doesn't let us get too much up in our heads and doesn't let our ego take over.

I truly do hate doing dishes, but I will only let them build up so much in the sink before I say, "Come on, Candy. Get it together. It's time to do the dishes." We can use this scenario in so many areas of our lives and with so many tasks. I'm sure you have one chosen already that fits in your own world.

Creating physical wellness also falls into a few different categories, especially when we talk about aging gracefully, those categories being cardiorespiratory wellness and musculoskeletal wellness. Basically, heart and lung strength and muscles and bone strength.

If we don't take care of our heart and lung health, then we will have trouble climbing stairs and walking a good distance as we get older. Now we might not give that any thought as we sit at our desks for eight hours a day, but as the years pass, this will become much more evident. That doesn't consider heart disease or lung disease that progressively comes with inactivity.

Our muscle and bone health are just as important. As we get older, it becomes more and more important to keep up with our bone health and muscle strength. As we age, our bone density, and therefore strength, begins to suffer. We need to work at maintaining our bone density not only with our diet but our exercise as well.

The same holds true for our muscle strength. As young as thirty years old, we start to lose 3–5 percent of our muscle strength per decade. So by the time we are seventy, we've quite possibly already lost 40 percent of our muscle strength just by aging. But that doesn't take into consideration that at the age of sixty-five, the rate increases to 8 percent per decade.

Clearly, we need to pay more attention to both our cardiorespiratory health and our musculoskeletal wellness now versus when we start to feel the decline in each of these areas. Prevention is always a better solution than reaction.

If we create consistent cardiovascular training along with an equally consistent resistance training practice, we can slow the aging process immensely. This doesn't mean you start training for a 5K and lifting large amounts of weight right out of the gate. That's the "Candy old way" of doing things, the all-in way, which almost never ends well. But it usually ends quickly. Hence the lack of consistency is a pattern.

When it comes to working out, the "all in" usually results in lots of DOMS or delayed-onset muscle soreness, which can quickly lead to a week or so of soreness that keeps you from doing any physical activity at all and, of course, not a good way to make progress.

You can start out on this part of your journey with a simple daily walk, whether that be outside in nature, on a treadmill in your basement, or at the gym. You can start with a short distance at a light pace and increase one or the other or both gradually. You can also choose any of several different kinds of cardio exercise as well.

The same can be done with resistance training. Resistance training comes in many different forms. You can use free weights, bands, body-weight exercises, and more.

Other things to be concerned with are flexibility and balance. As we age, our flexibility becomes more limited for several reasons, but mainly because of inflammation levels. Balance is another concern as our flexibility and strength dwindle. Balance and flexibility become more and more important as we age. Our muscles become weaker, and our bones become more brittle.

These are all great individual reasons to take better care of our physical health, but combined, they create some big hurdles to overcome. The key here is to start where you are and go at your own pace. I've spent too much time recovering from injuries and not making progress to continue in that all-or-nothing mindset. All it does is set us back and discourage us in the long run.

Starting where we are makes a huge difference, and progressing gradually can make so much more progress than you can ever imagine. We all have a different starting point. We all are on our own journey. Whether your priority is weight loss or building strength and longevity, it all has a different starting place and a different progression level.

That means we each need our own plan—our own workout regimen and routines and our own components to those routines. We each like something different. Some of us love to run, others despise it, and others just know their knees or hips or back won't take that kind of impact. That's the cool thing about it. Just like on our emotional and spiritual journey, we all have our own path, and it takes its own twists and turns along the way. The key is to just keep going and keep following that path wherever that may lead you.

My path has led me from lifting and running in my twenties to nothing and back. Then to yoga and qigong, then walking and hot yoga, HIIT workouts and walking, and now I'm lifting again and progressing from walking the dog back into running again. I'm just taking it a little more gradually this time around. My goals are long-term, and my focus is long-term as well.

Longevity and living a full life are my goals—feeling good and maximizing my energy throughout the rest of my life here on this planet. I also want to optimize the other areas of my wellness, creating the perfect balance of my emotional, spiritual, and physical wellness.

If this sounds great to you too, then ask yourself some of these questions to get started on the physical aspect of your overall well-being.

Where are you now physically? Is that where you want to be? Where do you want to be in twenty, thirty, and forty years or beyond? Where you are now, is that a possibility? What do you need to change to make that a reality? How do you begin? How will you progress? Do you need additional support? What does that look like?

These are some broad questions, but that is because they look different for each of us. I am a firm believer that we all need a coach. Some of us need them in one area versus another. I've had coaches in most areas of my life from one time to another.

What area do you feel you might need more help in? Let's face it—none of us are good at everything. We all need help somewhere, and that's nothing to be ashamed of. When we admit that and ask for help, that actually means we are strong enough to do so.

Ask yourself the above questions, sit down, and take some time to write out what you'd like to do, accomplish, and how you might get there. How can you progress on this path in a gradual manner that will not overwhelm you, burn you out, and land you in the healing chair for a week after you begin?

What activities are you passionate about and would like to get better at? Improve your skills, your time, and your strength, and find out how you will do that in a gradual but consistent way so as to never set yourself back. That's the key: gradual progression helps us get stronger a little bit at a time.

How will you show up? How often and is that enough to get you where you want to be? Keep your mind going and create the best scenario in your mind. Visualize this just like you did in our other two areas. How will it look, feel, and be in that moment as you are progressing on your physical wellness journey?

We have to enjoy what we do, so asking yourself these questions with that in mind is huge. Make sure you choose activities that you want to do, something that you enjoy participating in, and something that you aren't going to make excuses as to why you can't do them.

No matter what you choose, there will probably be days when your mind will want to do that anyway. Make excuses. I love my workouts and I know that I have to do them first thing in the morning, or they won't get done. But I still have those moments on many occasions where I don't want to get out of bed at 4:00 a.m. I don't want to lift and I don't want to go for a walk. I'm tired. I'd rather just go back to bed.

But I don't. I must push myself to do it anyway and keep doing it anyway. This morning, I didn't want to go for my walk in the rain, but I did. I put on the raincoat, grabbed the umbrella, and went anyway. I even ran for a few hundred feet, and tomorrow I plan to run a few hundred more. A little to a time so as to not have any back steps and injuries and ensure that I still enjoy what I'm doing.

I always take the time to recognize how much better I feel when I'm done with my workout on those days. It's so important to reinforce our actions with that end proof that says, "Yes, I'm glad I did push myself and I'm glad I did it anyway."

Then tomorrow morning when I'm not so sore that I can't get out of bed, I'll also be glad that I only ran a couple hundred feet, instead of what I used to do and regret pushing myself so far that I could barely get out of bed at all that day or the next or even the next. That's not fun, so why do we continue to do that to ourselves? Why do we continue to go down that all-or-nothing road?

That's why it has changed now. That does nothing but spin our wheels and set us back. From this point on, we will only make progress. As I proofread this manuscript, I'm reminded that some things are out of our control. I wrote this chapter several weeks ago. Right now, I sit here with a brace on my knee for a strained meniscus and MCL. Not because I pushed too much or ran too far but because while on one of our walks, Tobias went one way as I went another. My reactive pirouette wasn't nearly as graceful as I envisioned it to be.

This was clearly out of my control but is a good reminder of why we're doing this. So once again, we pivot. My rehab will take precedence, and my doctor advises cycling will be a better choice as my fifty-two-year-old knees are showing their wear. I used to love my spin classes, so I've invested in a bike for my gym. It comes this week. I'll just have to focus on pacing myself and healing at the start again.

18

BRINGING IT ALL TOGETHER

Alone we can do so little; together we can do so much.
—Helen Keller

At this point, we have visited all three pillars of our wellness: emotional, spiritual, and physical. Now we need to bring these three areas of our holistic wellness into balance with one another to create that truly balanced wellness we are looking for. This is where we've been missing the boat over time. We are always hyperfocused on one area over another because that is our nature, and we are all better at obsessing over one thing versus three.

We've taken the time in each section to be present with ourselves, our habits, and our own tendencies. If we've been honest with ourselves along the way, then we have a good inventory of what we want in our lives, what our deepest dreams are, and what we are willing to do to get them.

We've assessed our emotional state and brought up any of those emotional issues that we feel have held us back until now. We've dug into our spiritual wellness and analyzed our faith and our fears. We've finally come back to our physical selves and taken a good hard look at our physical wellness dreams and goals and what it will take to attain them.

Now our chore is to design a plan to bring it all into reality. So let's create an action plan to achieve all these goals and dreams in a way that is sustainable and progressive at the same time, no more fooling around. Will you join me? You can download my free workbook at www.candyholmesfoster.com/bonus/workbook.

When it comes to your emotional well-being, what are your biggest goals and dreams? What are our amazing spiritual goals and dreams? Finally, what are your physical goals and dreams? Take a sheet of paper or a notebook and write these dreams out in detail. You may need a page or more than one page for each. Take your time and stop when you feel it's just like you want it.

Now, take each one of these areas and reread what you've written. How long do you think it will take to attain this? Write it down. Do this with each of your pillars. When you're done with this step, come back to each of them again. One at a time, start to break it down into action steps. What needs to be done to achieve each of your pillar goals? Start with one and keep going until you are satisfied with what you have. Then you can move on to your next pillar.

Once you've completed this task, lay each of your goals out in front of you. Does it look possible to work on all three goals at the same time? Does your timeline need to change? What tools will you need along your journey to attain each of these goals? Do your three pillars make sense when placed side by side? Does one area need more attention than another? Does one need editing to feel good and cohesive with the other two? Does it feel like your life will be balanced and complete as a whole? Go back and work through this and make any corrections needed.

As you know, things will change along the way, but having a clear view of how you will attain your goals is a great place to start and get going with your inspired action with clarity and direction to keep you moving in the right direction. This process has allowed me to remove the overwhelmed state at the start of a project and kept me from wasting immense amounts of time wandering aimlessly instead of creating laser focus as to what I need to accomplish daily.

This process is very much like creating a business plan. In both cases, you need to assess the steps, monetary requirements, resources, and time needed to get each step done in a consistent and timely manner. Take the time to make this attainable one step at a time and then set your plans into action. Take that first step and then the next and the next and the next. You can do this. You can create these dreams one step at a time. And when the going gets tough, you can always fall back on your other pillars.

Your three pillars support each other as you move forward with each of them. So never leave one of them behind. You will need them all on this journey to your divine ascension. Follow your dreams and live your purpose according to your plan. Cocreate your own amazing life centered on your three pillars of holistic wellness.

With true balance emotionally, spiritually, and physically, you will be able to create all your dreams have to offer and better the world around you while you are at it. Remember if we weren't here to create our dreams, then why would we have them? Don't play small here. You are meant to be larger than life. It's time! It's time to face your fears and do it anyway. It's time to claim your dreams and take that very first, very bold action step and bring those dreams to fruition.

Your pillars will support each other when times get tough. When you are physically hurting, lean into your spiritual and emotional pillars. When you're emotionally compromised, allow your physical and spiritual pillars to take on the load. And when you have spiritual doubts (and we all do), fall back on your physical and emotional pillars to get you through and figure it out.

This journey was never proclaimed to be easy, but I'll bet money that it will be rewarding.

NOTES

1. Rebecca Campbell, *Work Your Light Oracle Cards* (Hay House UK Ltd., 2018). Trust the Niggle.
2. Alana Fairchild, *Isis Oracle* (Blue Angel Publishing, 2016). Isis oracle cards by Alana Fairchild. The card that I pulled was Abundance of Sothis. This card says, "Abundance in many forms is increasingly in flow to you. Continue your good work of building channels through which abundance can be delivered to you. Freely share your talents, love wisdom and self, and enjoy the abundance responsively flowing to you, in many forms, over and over again." This was a reminder for me to stop stressing about money and hours and to remember that I am always taken care of.
3. James Clear, *Atomic Habits* (Avery, an imprint of Penguin Random House, 2018). Habit Stacking.
4. https://pubs.niaaa.nih.gov, Alcohol commercials make up 1.5 percent of all advertisements on prime-time television and 7.0 percent of all advertisements in sports programming.
5. "Loving Kindness Meditation" https://www.nantien.org.au/
6. Adam Barralet and Vanessa Jean Boscarello Ovens, *Gifts of the Essential Oils* (Alchemy House Publishing, 2019).
7. Gabrielle Burnstein, The Universe Has Your Back, Hay House Inc. 2018
8. Maureen St. Germain, Beyond the Flower of Life. Bear & Company, Rochester, VT, 2009, 2021
9. Louise Hay, You Can Do It. Hay House Inc. 2021
10. Dr. Wayne Dyer, Excuses be Gone. Hay House Inc. 2011
11. Dr. Peter Attia MD, Outlive the science and art of longevity", Harmony Publishing 2023

ABOUT THE AUTHOR

Candy Holmes-Foster is a health coach, meditation instructor, and Reiki master teacher. The lessons she's learning on her journey to wellness have brought her to her purpose and her path. Candy is committed to sharing with the world the knowledge that there is no one way to find your true happiness and wellness.

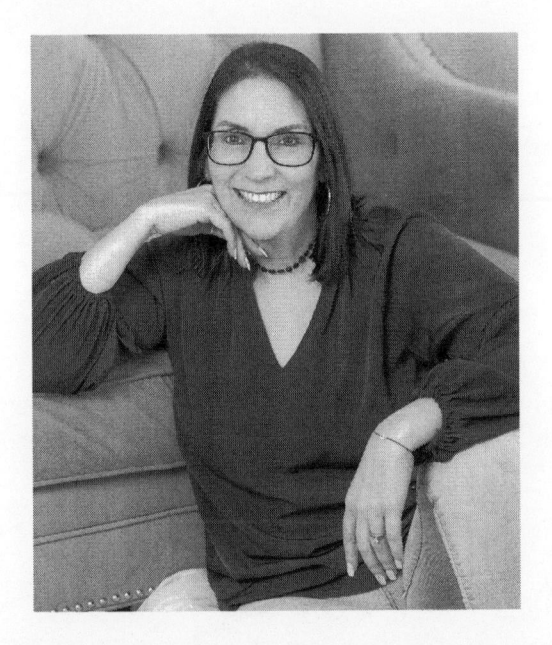

She is devoted to bringing meditation, Reiki, peace, love, and holistic wellness to the world and giving you back the power to create all of it in your own world. Candy believes we are all here to help each other thrive during this lifetime. Her part in this is helping you create your own version of holistic well-being and your own path to thrive on your journey.